praise for annie kay's work

"Marvelous! I was thrilled with the blend of weight management and yoga."

"Thank you so much for taking this subject out of the yoga closet. I know that my own awareness and compassion have increased tenfold."

"Annie is a wonderful, well-prepared presenter. This was presented in a compassionate Kripalu style. Thank you."

"Perfect in content and presentation. Annie brings her whole self into this work—very credible, grateful, and fun. Thanks so much."

"I thought this workshop really did a wonderful job of tying in self-acceptance, health rather than weight with the yoga benefits. Thank you!"

"Loved every bit of it! Many thanks for your presence, soothing voice, knowledge, and delivery. Excellent presentation."

"Profound—inspiring. Tons of good info. Amazingly strong and detailed."

"This was wonderful. Sane, intelligent, gentle, inspiring."

"Annie's workshop exceeded my expectations. Many profound insights. 'Self-love and self-care are our spiritual path to wholeness.' Thank you!"

"A wonderful blend of philosophy, science, strategies, and postures! I feel prepared to embark on a journey of my own—doing a workshop in my home studio. Thank you!"

"This program gave me great new ideas for having a healthier life. I deeply enjoyed this class."

"Annie was able to communicate such a positive approach to body image, to changing behaviors—it was very helpful. More!"

"You bring a grounded and loving energy to your work that allows each of us to take what we need. I would like to see women's groups on this."

how to have health, happiness...and a body you can live with and love

Our modern environment, filled with junk foods and empty calories, pushes us toward weight gain. At the same time we are inundated with media images that suggest we are failures if we aren't model thin. This culture of mixed messages undermines our ability to be happy with who we are.

That's where *Every Bite Is Divine* shines. Its essential message is that we each have a perfect natural weight and shape. By remembering how to care for ourselves lovingly, we allow ourselves to gracefully create our unique and healthy body. Crash diets are not in this picture. Through yoga and other methods of relaxation and rediscovering our individual self-care basics, we can find our true self. We can enjoy life—including eating as we love to eat—and reach a healthy contentment with our own reality even if it doesn't match the picture popular culture sells.

Explore why *Every Bite Is Divine*, and discover:

- Why diets put your mind and body in the mode to *gain*, not lose, weight—and simple ways to reverse the trend

- How you are continually bombarded with cues to eat exactly what's wrong for you—and how you can inoculate yourself

- When "fight or flight" turns into "stew and chew." You can short-circuit the cycle, manage stress—and drop pounds the healthy way

Avoid being a casualty in the collision between human biology and modern society. *Every Bite Is Divine* puts you on the path to finding balance and stretching joyfully, confidently, and contentedly into loving who you really are.

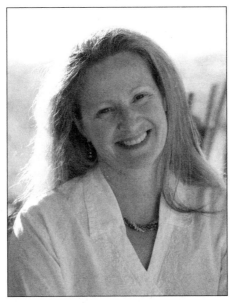

Photo by Terry Pommett

ANNIE B. KAY, MS, RD, RYT, is a unique voice as a writer, speaker, spokesperson, and teacher. Her rare blend of scientific education in nutrition, practical training in yoga, and her personal health story brings unusual dimension to her endeavors in communicating the art and science of health. Annie is a graduate of Cornell University (nutritional biochemistry) and Boston University (nutrition communications) and has numerous scientific papers to her credit. She has written for *Cooking Light,* among other national magazines, and has appeared on CNN and in the national media on topics of health and wellness. Annie has integrated leading-edge information on how the body works with her experience practicing and teaching yoga to develop an innovative approach to cultivating awareness, mind-body balance, and weight normalization. Annie lives on Nantucket Island, MA, and on the island of Kauai, HI. She lives with her surfer husband, Craig, and her crazy cat, Rahu. In addition to writing, speaking, and teaching, Annie is a home chef, gardener, and poet dedicated to creativity, service, and fun.

every bite is divine

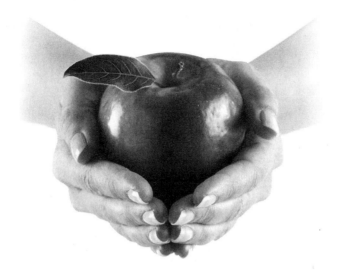

every bite is divine

The balanced approach to enjoying eating,
feeling healthy and happy, and getting to
a weight that's natural for you

annie b. kay, MS, RD, RYT

*Life
Arts* PRESS

CAMBRIDGE, MA 02139

every bite is divine

The balanced approach to enjoying eating, feeling healthy
and happy, and getting to a weight that's natural for you

Life Arts PRESS

CAMBRIDGE, MA 02139 • www.lifeartspress.com

--- Publisher's Cataloguing-in-Publication ---

Kay, Annie B.
　　Every bite is divine : the balanced approach to enjoying eating,
　　feeling healthy and happy, and getting to a weight that's natural for you /
　　by Annie B. Kay. — 1st ed. — Cambridge, MA : Life Arts Press, 2007.

　　　　p. ; cm.
　　　　(Every bite is divine)

　　　　ISBN-13: 978-0-9787438-3-3
　　　　Includes bibliographical references and index.

　　　　1. Weight loss. 2. Weight loss—Psychological aspects. 3. Food habits.
　　　　4. Body weight—Psychological aspects. 5. Self-actualization (Psychology)
　　　　6. Yoga. I. Title.

　　RM222.2 .K39 2007　　　　　　　　　　　　　　2006906192
　　613.2/5--dc22　　　　　　　　　　　　　　　　0701

*This book is intended as a supplement to, not a replacement for, regular medical care. The
information provided here is intended to help you make informed decisions about your
health. Talk to your doctor before adopting this or any other health regimen. If you suspect
that you have a medical problem, please seek competent medical care immediately.*

Permissions and appreciations appear on page 163.

Life Arts Press is an enthusiastic member of the Green Press Initiative, and adheres to
their guidelines on the use of recycled papers.

Book Design: Peri Poloni-Gabriel, Knockout Design, www.knockoutbooks.com
Book Editor: Brookes Nohlgren, Books by Brookes, booksbybrookes@earthlink.net
Book Consultant: Ellen Reid, Ellen Reid's Book Shepherding, www.bookshep.com

Printed in the United States of America.

For Margaret and Stanley Barry,

who somehow gave six of us just the start in life we needed.

This book is in honor of you, with love and gratitude.

contents

acknowledgments

Like any worthwhile project, this one is the product of many talented minds and hands. Special thanks to Ellen Reid and the stellar creative and editorial team she pulled together for this project: Laren Bright, Peri Poloni-Gabriel, Jennifer Repo, Brookes Nohlgren, and Natalie Giboney. Ellen's expertise, kindness, and passion for the work were absolutely critical to its coming into being. Her talented and creative crew each had a hand in making *Every Bite Is Divine* as beautiful and inspiring as it is. Thanks also to artist Kevin Hughes, who developed our yoga illustrations, and Terry Pommett for photos.

Appreciation goes to Wolf Rinke and his team for their work on and support of the clinical course *Yoga and Meditation: Tools for Weight Management,* which preceded *Every Bite Is Divine.* I also send gratitude to my friends and colleagues who thoughtfully reviewed earlier versions of this work: Christina Economos, PhD; Kristann Hentz, MD; Liz Weiss, MS, RD; Bonita Oelke, MS, RD; Francesca Vanegas; Shirley Pantoliano, MS, RD; Kathianne Sellars, MEd, RD, LDN, CSCS; Stephanie Vangsness, MS, RD, LDN, CNSD; and Caitlin Hosmer, MS, RD.

My very deepest gratitude goes to the master teachers at Kripalu and to master yoginis and teachers Barbara Benagh and Silvia Bhavani Maki for the indelible impression they have made on my practice, my teaching, and my life. I am also always grateful to my ever-curious and buoyant colleagues at the Yoga Room on Nantucket: Paul Bruno, Bettina Broer, Natasha Foy, Michael Rich, and yogini Shannah Green, whose grace created the space and keeps it together.

Thanks to the individuals who have experienced my work and responded enthusiastically. I'm honored to have witnessed your efforts, and your experience has made me a better teacher.

And finally, thanks to my beloved husband and partner, Craig Kay, who didn't volunteer to live every detail of the long and arduous process of birthing a book, but did, with his usually open heart, light and generous spirit, and love. Lucky me.

introduction

When the pupil is ready, the teacher appears.

— YOGI RAMACHARAKA

My body and I have had a turbulent relationship.

Some of my earliest memories are of racing through the fragrant pine forest behind my house, crawling through the underbrush to scout the best site for the girls' tree fort. We played tomboy games of escape in the summer twilight. I reveled in movement. I enjoyed my body with the enthusiasm of discovery and the pride of ownership. But somewhere along the line that early joy was squelched. A dissonance grew between what I saw as the realities of my female physical body, the changing emotional needs of my heart, and the thoughts and beliefs of my teenage mind.

I was in an early wave of the generation that Mary Pipher, PhD, describes so well in her book *Reviving Ophelia*. Girls who experienced a disconnect from themselves as they came of age. As I grew through adolescence I lost track of those things I loved, including my passions for physicality, art, and nature. I focused instead on being what others (my classmates, boys, and the evermore ubiquitous media) seemed to want and expect me to be. I grew up in the '60s and '70s watching media images of beauty grow super thin, culminating in Twiggy and heroin chic. Oh, the titillating shock of extreme thinness! And I liked it. And I could do it. Almost. The only problem was that a full social life required eating, and lots of it. So many thin girls seemed to be able to eat cheeseburgers, fries, Cokes, and never gain weight. It just didn't add up.

I remember my freshman biology teacher introducing the idea of women who vomited after gorging on junk food. The women who did this were presented as selfish, crazy, and bad Christians, but a seed was sewn in my mind. Though it was "bad," here was an easy solution to an impossible problem. So I began to experiment. And it worked. At first, purging was an occasional way to deal with high-calorie social situations. But it kept expanding. It made me feel more in control, even though a world of deceit and secrecy was wrapped around it and I often felt physically lousy because of it. It became a larger and larger part of my life. By the time I was a sophomore in high school, I had a full-blown eating disorder. While I eventually got the guidance and support I needed to end the destructive cycle, disordered eating and its emotional paradigm haunt me to this day. Certainly the consumer culture and media obsession with super-thinness haven't changed. The unhealthy trends that promote eating more and faster and doing more in less time haven't changed. But who I am and how I care for myself have.

My passion for food and the body was fed as I studied nutrition at Cornell and Boston University, cooking my way through school in restaurants as varied as the health food co-op to the five-star white linen bistro. I reveled in the sensuality of the dining experience. *And I struggled with weight and eating.* I wrote about food. I developed healthy and delicious recipes for books and websites. *And I struggled with weight and eating.* I worked as a clinician, encountering people who suffer the chronic health consequences of lifetimes of overabundance, or the deprivation of body-wasting diseases. *And I struggled with weight and eating.*

Through my work I noticed that even those whose lives depend upon making dietary changes often cannot do it. Living a healthy lifestyle is much more than knowing what to eat. By the time most of us hit 40, our dietary patterns and our bodies reflect years of emotional and physical life. I have counseled women trapped in a diet-binge cycle. They have come to me with a hatred for their bodies that set the stage for compulsive eating and unhappy lives. I know others who have starved themselves for years and are fashionably thin but have malnourished bodies and sad, deprived spirits. I know many men and women who have struck a dynamic balance between enjoying food and maintaining their weight; each of them has written their own equation for how that balance works. How and what we eat reflect how we feel about ourselves on the deepest of levels. And eating is one of life's greatest sensual experiences. But finding and keeping the balance of eating well, sustaining health through times of stress, and enjoying food without compulsion is, for many, one of modern life's great struggles. And it simply doesn't have to be.

When I was 32, I ended a difficult 10-year relationship. There is a saying in yoga, "When the student is ready the teacher appears." Yoga came to me at a time of personal transition and seeking. I was single and on my own for the first time in my adult life. Thanks to yoga, for perhaps the first time since childhood, I loved my entire body and didn't care if it was picture perfect. I found focus, balance, and strength, and remembered who I was under all that need I had to be beautiful and successful. That's when my own reality project— experiencing judgment-free glimpses of who I am and how to tend myself—began.

As I traveled inward, science marched on. A revolution in the science of nutrition was underway, and the body of research around weight management was growing. New behavioral approaches to weight loss deemphasizing dieting and supporting the adoption of long-term habits were gaining popularity and legitimacy. I found that looking at the new science through the paradigm of yoga worked, and I began to introduce it into my nutrition practice. My patients responded with relief and enthusiasm. They began to care for themselves compassionately, reconnecting with themselves and their passions rather than continuing to bury their emotions under eating and deprivation as they tried to be someone they were not. And they responded by achieving their realistic nutritional goals more easily—getting healthier and getting happier. You will hear their thoughts and stories reflected in the fictional characters I've created to help illustrate the *Every Bite Is Divine* process.

Yoga is much more than physical exercise, though it is certainly that. It can help you to slow down enough to appreciate the sweetness of the present moment and everything in it. Even, and especially, you. It fosters something that so many of us don't have nearly enough of in our bustling, striving lives: contentment (santosa*).

A central part of yoga is its ethical framework—its guidelines for living. Yogic principles include truth (satya*), non-violence (ahimsa*), purity and simplification (saucha*). We all sense that these are good, if abstract, principles to live by. Variations echo through many religious and spiritual practices. Contemplating these tenets while exploring the physical interplay of strength, will, flexibility, and surrender in our own body provides a context that makes them personal and meaningful. And those who struggle with body weight and a healthy

* Sanskrit terms discussed in depth in Chapter Two: Yoga and Meditation: An Alchemy of Awareness.

4

body image can explore these issues through yoga within a highly personal, relevant, and compassionate paradigm. Conscious eating is yoga at the table—we can explore the same issues by simply paying attention to and enjoying the process of nourishment. At the end of the day, yoga is about remembering the reality of who you are and finding both wonder and contentment in that.

There is a growing body of Western science investigating how yoga works. We will explore the fascinating science that reveals the interplay of respiration (breathing) and emotion, and the science behind the power of the mind to heal. The ancient Indian spiritual practice of yoga may be the missing piece in the puzzle of how to take care of yourself cohesively. After years of disunion, you can reintroduce your physical, emotional, and spiritual selves to one another through the practice of yoga.

This book is a culmination of a lifetime of personal experience and professional training. Considering diet and weight through the compassionate context of yoga worked for me in a way that other diets and strategies did not. It was a tool for rediscovering, and then reconnecting with, an authentic self and with authentic movement—how to *be* in my body. From that understanding, the re-learning of basic self-care founded on real physical and emotional needs could evolve. Expanding yoga's gifts to diet and self-care can be an antidote to our culture's unhealthy media bombardment that is in large part aimed at women but sprays us all. It can be an antidote to the unhealthy diet and weight loss industry, and to the fashion media who feed the need for thinness. As you remember and deepen your reality project through the practice of yoga and eating awareness, you may begin to develop immunity to the unrealistic messages that surround you. You will begin to recognize that consumerism is not going to feed or complete you. These compulsive messages simply will no longer apply to you.

I also wrote this book to add my voice to the healthy weight fray. Indeed, I'm hoping that my voice adds to the sanity rather than the chaos of the weight loss industry. Over and over in my professional life I have seen individuals working in earnest to improve their lives by improving their health. And more often than not, people's positive motivation to improve their health is subverted. There is so much misinformation that sounds so true! Some self-proclaimed experts misinform for financial or ego expansion; some out of naïveté. I have spent much of my life working to be a balanced voice of reason, simplicity, and sanity.

Every Bite Is Divine is more than just another diet book. It's a compassionate framework through which to view not only what you eat, but also how you feel and who you are. It's a whole lifestyle book. No lists of denied foods or needless sacrifices. Just conscious choices and a process for making them. For those of us with weight and eating issues, learning to care for our bodies with love and compassion and without compulsion is part of our lifelong spiritual path. I hope to grow a community of support for all of us who share that path.

Every Bite Is Divine aims for the root of the problem of weight—the underlying issues that are causing you to overeat and preventing you from moving. Then, rather than forcing you into a diet that works for *others*, it provides personal, gradual, doable suggestions for making lasting and permanent changes that work for *you*. *Every Bite Is Divine* is based on the latest nutrition, behavioral, and movement science and acknowledges from day one that change is not easy, but it is something you can do for yourself in order to live your fullest life.

Every Bite Is Divine is a tool to help you achieve a healthy weight for your age, body frame size, and lifestyle. This book can't lose weight for you. But it will help you understand the internal and external environments that make you gain weight. It can't make you into someone you are not and were never meant to be. But it can be a key to help you unlock the beauty and perfection of your truest self.

Perhaps *Every Bite Is Divine* will touch you with a means of coming home to your heart and to your truth. Buddhists say that life is essentially suffering through self-inflicted illusions. But to me (and to them), there is also boundless happiness and joy. You can face the inevitable drawbacks and suffering of life with grace and an open heart. That open heart can access the transcendent joy that is right in front of you, and right inside of you.

That is what I wish for you.

Namaste ("The divinity within me
bows to the divinity within you"),

annie

prologue

THE WORM'S WAKING

*This is how a human can change: there's a worm addicted
to eating grape leaves.*

*Suddenly, he wakes up, call it grace, whatever, something
wakes him, and he's no longer a worm.*

*He's the entire vineyard, and the orchard too, the fruit, the trunks,
a growing wisdom and joy that doesn't need to devour.*

— RUMI

Barbara exhaled. Natural light and the lilt of soft piano music flowed through the room. Several blue yoga mats topped with velour cushions faced a lacquered vase holding a single orchid. Another cushion sat up front. She let her shoulders drop as she stood in the studio's foyer and felt the relief of release. At the very least, she thought, I can relax in this room. With her friend Suzanne, Barbara had signed up for my workshop called East-West Weight Management, and both of them had kept their expectations in check. Barbara's main concern was the possibility of breaking a sweat, which she usually artfully avoided. She really wasn't into exercise, and she knew that was part of why, at 53, she weighed 240 pounds and had cholesterol and blood pressure readings that raised the eyebrows of her doctor and nurses more alarmingly with each annual physical. Barbara works at the local home center, behind the counter and supervising the summer workers that flow into town. She is married to Skip, a third-generation fisherman and a red-nosed meat-and-potatoes man. Anything she cooks with vegetables gets the stink-eye from Skip.

Suzanne works in the rough-and-tumble world of local real estate. Her days consist of driving the town from dawn to dusk, cell phone grafted to ear. She lunches with wealthy urbanites hoping to find a peaceful escape while simultaneously making a killing in the region's eternally hot market. She's the one to make their dreams come true, *now*. Suzanne used to enjoy the fast-paced life more but, at 46, she wonders if the tension is catching up with her. Lately, she feels achy all the time and has noticed that while she has always been slim she is developing an inner tube of thickness around her belly. She has noticed that her weight has been creeping up over the last few years, and she now carries 138 pounds on her petite frame; she'd always been about 125 and never needed to do much about her weight. She has also just received her first high blood pressure score, so she is thinking about how to take better care of herself. Suzanne is married to another real estate professional. Her husband is fit, conscientious about his health, and revels in the high-pressure life. They attend all the socially important fundraisers in town and are often seen dining out with friends.

A young woman with brown hair swinging bounces into the studio. Christine moved to town with a boyfriend after college, and stayed when he left. She works in the restaurant trade, which is fast paced and then dead, high pressure then dead. The restaurant crowd is a social one and Christine often joins them for late-night drinks at local bars. Since her high school days Christine, now 34, has struggled with an eating disorder. Bulimia sounds clinical and unreal to her, but she knows that's a category she occupies, and she knows it's not good. It seems to be the only way she's maintained her normal weight of 128 pounds for her medium frame. Several times each week she binges on bowl after bowl of cereal or ice cream, or something else that's creamy and comforting, and then purges by vomiting. She has no idea why she does it, but she often feels physically horrible but curiously relieved afterwards. At times it seems to go away, but for whatever reason it always creeps back.

A sandy-haired man lumbers in. Tom used to be a surfer but now he mostly watches. The same with work—he used to be a carpenter, but now that he's a general contractor, he does more oversight than swinging of hammers. His body has thickened in the middle as he's taken to the sidelines. His weight has steadily climbed to his latest high of 286 pounds on his 6-foot frame. He knew that he'd been steadily gaining weight, but the number on the scale shocked and panicked him. He hates the way he looks, but may hate even more the thought of kicking the TV, beer, and chips habit on nights and weekends that is his one escape and source of comfort from his long days and busy family life. Tom's father died when he was about Tom's age of 55, and when Tom looks in the mirror he sees his dad.

Anita entered the studio and gave a little wave to Barbara and Suzanne, family friends. Anita has been big all her life. At 28, she weighs 320 pounds, and doesn't know if that's bad or really bad, or what to do about it. She was recently diagnosed with type 2 diabetes and is just beginning to learn what that means. A dietitian at the local hospital suggested that she try this workshop as a way of exploring her eating and other lifestyle habits. Anita knows that she's probably never going to be thin, and she can come to terms with that, though she frankly wonders if her family can. She just hopes to look her best and be healthy. Anita is an attorney, and until recently worked in a prestigious firm in New York. In the last year, she'd been passed over for three promotions while she knows she was the best young lawyer in her firm. Anita has recently moved home for a year and is working at a local legal office to "get her life together," which includes getting a handle on her weight and health.

"Welcome to the workshop. I'm Annie," I say.

Each class member is happy to see a personable, average-appearing woman rather than a super-thin, wrinkle-free rubber band. "Just leave your shoes and personal things in the dressing room, and come on in. There are chairs for those of you not comfortable getting up and down from the floor. Let's begin."

Anita, Barbara, Suzanne, Christine, and Tom follow me into the room, nodding greetings to one another as they each find a place. They take a seat, settle in, and settle down.

chapter one

the obesity epidemic: national trends, personal stories

*It is no measure of health to be well adjusted
to a profoundly sick society.*

— KRISHNAMURTI

An epidemic? It sounds so distant and abstract, doesn't it? But it's not. It's on every street corner and in every school, in every town in America. Each of our workshop participants has a personal version of this country's obesity problem. You may too. If you feel like Barbara, you're not alone. By any measure, obesity in America, and around the world, has exploded.

Every one of us has a unique profile of numbers and factors in our lives that make up an equation that results in our body weight. There are national trends and cultural shifts that underlie

"I just don't recognize myself anymore," said Barbara during our first meeting. "I can't see myself inside my physical body, but I don't recognize who I've become either. I used to be more fun and liked myself better. But now I feel lost inside all the things that make up my life — kids, work. Food is my solace, and it shows."

the epidemic of weight gain that so many of us experience. Our modern world loads the weight-gain end of that equation. Learning your own personal equation is the first step to balancing it and managing your weight.

So, just how overweight are we?

Very. Between 1960 and 1980, Americans gradually gained weight, and obesity numbers began to rise. But since 1980, that trend has skyrocketed. Recent national data shows that 65% of U.S. adults—over 192 million people—are overweight. The proportion of children who are overweight has also exploded and is triple the rate it was in 1980.

Most Modern Roads Lead to Weight Gain

Weight gain usually doesn't happen overnight, but develops over decades. It's the bottom-line result of years of small decisions, many of them unconscious, that you make throughout each day. Snappy, simple solutions, despite what you hear in the media, just don't exist. As our workshop participants share their experiences about the factors that have tipped their weight gain equation, perhaps your own weight story will begin to become clear.

The forgotten magic of movement

Modern technology has transformed our lives. The wonders of automation now make it possible to lead a full and productive life—to work, shop, talk to friends, and be entertained without moving from the comfort of the couch. Kids play video games rather than playing outside after school. And our time spent watching TV continues to rise. The result of all this technological improvement? Today, at every

Energy In: What Are Americans Eating?

Across the country, a large jump in the calories we eat happened between 1985 and 2000, without a corresponding increase in calories burned through physical activity. Now, Americans eat way more fat, sugar, and processed grains than we used to. You can see how much our intake exceeds recommendations in Charts 1 and 2 below. According to national data, Americans may be eating up to twice the calories they need to in order to maintain their body weight.

Chart 1: Added Fat (65) vs. Recommendations (41)

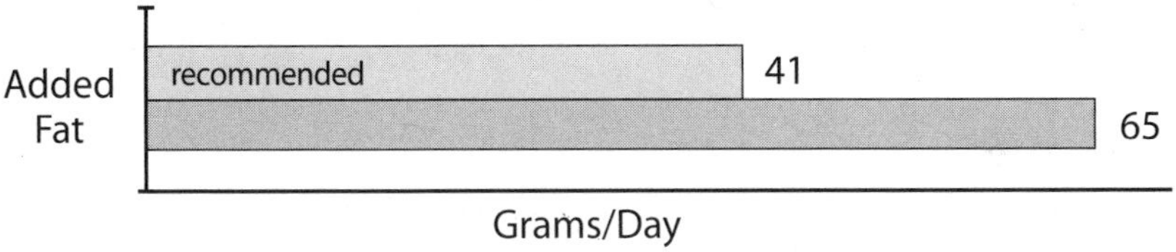

Added Fat
- recommended — 41
- 65

Grams/Day

Chart 2: Added Sugar (31) vs. Recommendations (12)

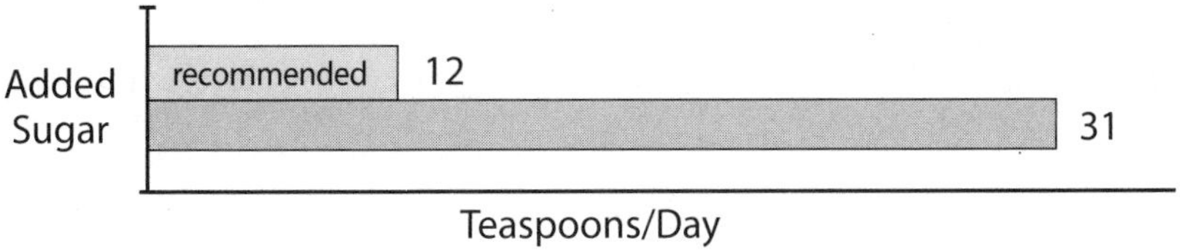

Added Sugar
- recommended — 12
- 31

Teaspoons/Day

Source: Economic Research Service, *FoodReview*, Vol 25 Issue 3, Winter 2002.

stage of life, Americans are less active. According to national surveys, half of Americans do not meet national recommendations for physical activity, and almost one-quarter of adults report no leisure time physical activity at all.

What is moderate activity? Walking, washing the car, vacuuming, and gardening are just a few examples. More are outlined in Chart 3. The Surgeon General (our nation's doctor) says that "every American

"I can see that shift," said Barbara. "When I was in school, almost everyone walked." The others nodded. "Now, 'walkers' almost don't exist—every kid takes the bus. Safety and schedules just warrant rides. And you know, transportation wasn't the only thing that was more physical. My mother was always physically on the move, cleaning the house and preparing meals without all the electrical appliances I have. I can't say life was better. But it was more physical than mine today."

can benefit from 30 minutes of moderate activity on most, if not all, days of the week." Nearly any physical movement counts. More activity, like moving for a longer period of time, or more vigorously, can lead to even greater benefits. An active life is not just for the fit and the beautiful—it's for *every single one* of us, no matter your size, your sex, your physical ability, or the size of your bank account. If you are in a wheelchair, wheel and you'll have health benefits. Chart 3 shows some basic activities that will burn at least a very minimum of 100 calories. Do one of these five times each week and you will meet the national recommendation for health.

Movement changes your body and your mind for the better from the inside out. Nearly every aspect of your body works better when you are active. Exercise has been shown to be as effective as anti-depressant medication in treating mild depression. And best of all, physical activity can boost your metabolism. It's like changing your body from a 2-cylinder to a V-8.

Anita found the message of moderate physical activity good news. "Now that I am finally ready to really pay attention to my body," she said, "one of the first things I've heard is that moderate activity—just walking more—could be a good first step. I am not one for spandex! Since I've started to be more active, I've felt better and looked better—almost immediately. For me, physical activity is key."

Chart 3: Examples of Moderate Physical Activity (100-200 Calories)

Common Chores	Sporting Activities
Washing and waxing a car for 45-60 minutes	Playing volleyball for 45-60 minutes
Washing windows or floors for 45-60 minutes	Playing touch football for 45 minutes
Gardening for 30-45 minutes	Walking 1¾ miles in 35 minutes (20 min/mile)
Wheeling self in wheelchair for 30-40 minutes	Basketball (shooting baskets) for 30 minutes
Pushing a stroller 1½ miles in 30 minutes	Bicycling 5 miles in 30 minutes
Raking leaves for 30 minutes	Dancing fast (social) for 30 minutes
Walking 2 miles in 30 minutes (15 min/mile)	Water aerobics for 30 minutes
Shoveling snow for 15 minutes	Swimming laps for 20 minutes
Stair walking for 15 minutes	Basketball (playing game) for 15-20 minutes
	Bicycling 4 miles in 15 minutes
	Jumping rope for 15 minutes
	Running 1½ miles in 15 minutes (10 min/mile)

Source: U.S. Surgeon General's Report on Physical Activity and Health, 1996.

Tom once said to me, "When I think about it, I live in doughnut-land. I eat what's there, and what's there is junk food. In my car, at work, the kitchen counters at home—junk. I've never really thought about changing that. It would be an adjustment, no doubt, but if fruit were around or really there looking at me, I'd probably eat more of that."

Does your environment endanger your weight-health?

Health doesn't blossom in a vacuum. Your surroundings profoundly impact your health decisions, and those decisions are made within the environments of your home, workplace, and community. For example, you may choose not to walk to the store or work because of a lack of sidewalks. If fresh fruit is five days old and buried in the back of the refrigerator, but the chocolate cake is right out on the counter, what are you going to grab for a quick snack? With fewer options for physical activity and healthy eating, it becomes more difficult for us to make healthy choices. Time spent taking control of your environment and making simple adjustments can ease your path toward tipping your weight equation in a healthy direction. Chart 4 may give you some ideas for those environmental shifts. Begin with those that seem easiest.

Genetics and health history: Your weight legacy

Some of us inherit a predisposition toward obesity. But inheriting a predisposition is not a sure life sentence for obesity. Genotype influence

"I have been overweight all my life," said Anita. "And both my parents are too. Maybe there is a genetic factor involved, but I know that anything I've learned about how to be healthy, well, my family pretty much does the opposite. I love my mom's food, but it's like the list of things not to eat if you want to be a healthy weight—fried chicken, French fries, creamy dressings, serious desserts. And athletic? Don't even think about it. If I do get healthier, I'll be a real trailblazer in my family!"

Chart 4: Remodel Your Environment to Enhance Energy Balance

Location	Remodeling Idea
Home	• Reduce time spent watching TV and in other sedentary behaviors—try meditating, or other evening rituals, to relax. • Build physical activity into regular routines such as cleaning and other household chores. • "Sell" yourself and your family healthy food choices by showcasing them in a place they are easily seen in the refrigerator, on kitchen counters, etc. • Get rid of candy dishes except for special occasions. Replace them with flowers or something that will give you a visual lift. • Keep a list of ideas for physical activity or your health goals somewhere you will see them every day.
Work	• Again, lose the candy dishes. Is there something like flowers, or a hand-squeeze toy, that can help you to ease stress? • Take the stairs rather than the elevators. • How can you increase your movement throughout your workday? Disco breaks? Brief walks at lunchtime?

on our weight is greatly impacted by our behavior, environment, and other things we've discussed, such as abundant food supply or little physical activity.

Some illnesses may lead to weight gain. These include Cushing's disease and polycystic ovary syndrome. And many drugs, including steroids and some antidepressants, may also cause weight gain. These things may make losing weight a challenge, but they may also be motivators to encourage you. Who more than you deserves to be well cared for? No one.

The mind-body cost of convenience

Food is big business, and we all experience the nutritional fallout from an increasingly commercialized food supply. If you are an average American, you are exposed to at least 3,000 advertisements every day and will spend three years of your life watching TV commercials. Most of us claim not to pay attention to advertising, and both consumers and advertisers claim that advertising does not influence what we buy. The billions spent on advertising by corporations, however, strongly suggests otherwise. We have all heard about the strong relationship between children watching televised food advertising and their diets ending up featuring the advertised foods. Ninety-five percent of food ads in children's programming are for four cheap-to-produce food categories: soft drinks, candy, fast food, and sugar-coated cereals.

How do ads and media messages that our conscious mind knows are untrue influence us? According to Rance Crain, former editor-in-chief of *Advertising Age,* "Only eight percent of an ad's message is received by the conscious mind; the rest is worked and reworked deep within the recesses of the brain, where a product's positioning and repositioning takes shape." Researcher and consumer advocate Jean Kilbourn notes that it is in this sense that advertising is subliminal— not in the sense of hidden messages, but in the sense that individuals are not consciously aware of what advertising does. The advertising industry is filled with smart and sophisticated people who expertly craft messages that link our deepest emotions to commercial products. Those who struggle with weight and eating face a particularly strong current of unhealthy media projections from the cultural phenomenon of the cult of thinness.

The cult of thinness

The ever-present media's shouts and whispers have built a slim yet voluptuous beauty ideal in most of our minds. For the vast majority of women, however, the media's beauty ideal is impossible to attain. In the video *Slim Hopes*, researcher Jean Kilbourn notes that failure to achieve the beauty ideal is inevitable, even for models and actresses whose images are retouched and imperfections airbrushed away. Literally no one can be that perfect! It seems that the media purposefully undermines our inherent sense that we are OK as we are. Media images seem intent on encouraging us to break our own hearts through self-criticism. Study after study finds that most of us feel horrible about our own bodies. And what is the solution to the heartbreak of never measuring up to the culture's definition of beauty? If you look to the media for cues, it's shop or eat. Dysfunctional eating (and its couch-potato lifestyle counterparts) happens when emotions that make you feel weak or less-than-OK determine what you eat. It's when your basest fears rule what you do. The media culture reinforces these emotions because having dysfunctional lifestyles makes us great consumers for quick-fix fad diets, gourmet ice cream, cosmetic surgery, and whatever else is offered as the salve for our emotional wounds.

"I've always loved fashion, loved fashion magazines," said Christine. *"And it's important to me to look great. That means being slim. But do I feel great? Definitely not... I've been on a diet as far back as I can remember. But when I look back at pictures, I was so slim! If I could only have been happy and confident of my looks then. What a waste!"*

> As we talked about some of the issues common for eating disorders, Christine lit up. "I never really thought of my eating disorder as the way I deal with strong emotions, but that may be what I do. And, I notice that my eating is worse when I'm tired. This is the first time I've really put that together."

Food and beauty ads in particular are both beguiling and outright deceptive, and often normalize or glamorize dangerous attitudes toward eating. Women's magazines are peppered with articles on how to lose weight quickly, alongside ads for double chocolate cakes. Potato chips carry labels of "no cholesterol," and cereals whose content is 50% sugar sit with orange juice and an egg and claim "part of this nutritious breakfast." These claims and accompanying deceptive imagery and moralistic language muddy the waters of your ability to gather information you need to choose a healthy diet, and do no favors to your body image. Many people, understandably, just give up.

Good News: Times *Are* Changing

There is a movement toward healthier ads featuring normal women realistically portrayed. Nike, Dove, and others have undertaken advertising strategies to reinforce positive emotions in women.

Disordered eating

In the United States, as many as 10 million women and girls, and 1 million men and boys, have eating disorders. People with eating disorders tend to share a sense of overwhelming ineffectiveness. Every eating disorder begins with a diet. But, sometimes, the diet takes over. A vicious cycle of dieting spirals out of control in an attempt to gain self-control over weight. Difficulties in feeling inner sensations and a struggle with understanding and tolerating strong emotions are also central features of eating disorders.

The weight-loss circus

Until recently, dieting has been considered by obesity researchers and nutritionists a one-way ticket to gaining weight. That went double if you are a woman, and triple if you are a woman over 40. However, recent science has brought this idea of cycling (a never-ending spiraling of weight for chronic dieters) into question. But cycling may not be quite the endless weight-gain trap as often as suspected. This is good news for the chronic dieter in that it is always worthwhile to make the effort to lead a healthier life. Trying will not always backfire into more weight. It's important, however, that you summon your discriminatory powers so that you can resist the siren songs of quick-fix fads and choose a sound plan to real health. That's the secret to stepping out of the spiral for good.

The number of people diagnosed with eating disorders remains relatively small. But because of the secretiveness and shame associated with eating disorders, many cases may not be reported. A much greater percentage of the population, and particularly women, struggles with a hatred of their bodies and sub-clinical disordered eating attitudes and behaviors. These pervasive attitudes and behaviors lay the foundation for unhealthy dieting that can lead to disordered eating patterns.

"I've always said that my weight didn't really bother me," said Anita. "But of course deep down it does. My own obese mother says she's proud of me, but she also said that as long as I'm fat my achievements won't mean anything. And I wonder if my weight had something to do with my not getting the promotions I know I deserved. I thought I was doing well by not internalizing all these 'be thin' messages, but I do wonder if all anyone can see is my weight."

Body image

Your body image is your internal emotional response to your own body size and appearance. For many individuals, self-esteem (the value you place on yourself) is intimately intertwined with your positive or negative body image. A negative body image often increases with increased weight. A recent survey found that 77% of normal-weight college women wanted to lose weight. Moreover, 59% of the sample selected a target weight in the underweight range. These normal-weight women desired a body weight that was thin to the point of being unhealthy! When you are dissatisfied with your body weight, you are more likely to indulge in weight-control behaviors. And every eating disorder begins with a weight-loss diet.

"I am always on the go," said Suzanne as we shared our daily stress experiences. "I used to enjoy it, but I have to say the hustle and jostle of real estate is wearing on me. I don't have to work as much as I used to, but I just don't seem to know how to slow down. What would I do with myself?"

The stress connection

If nutritionally empty food and lack of activity are not enough to trigger weight gain, the spiral of stress can tip the scales. You are bombarded every day with life events, large and small, that trigger your body's stress response. Unfortunately, the design of your body does not take into account the nature of today's stress and our modern response to stressful events. When your body encounters a potentially dangerous situation—be it real, potential, or imagined—hormones are released that trigger your "fight or flight" response. Your heart rate increases, digestion slows, pupils dilate, and blood flow lessens to the limbs, all to prepare for the upcoming battle or escape.

The glitch comes with our modern response to the activation of our "fight or flight" response to stress. When, for example, your boss makes an unreasonable demand, do you prepare to do physical battle? Punch her in the nose? Make a mad dash for the door? Probably not. Most of us either stew or redirect our frustration. Unfortunately, your body doesn't recognize stewing as a reasonable response to stress, so the "fight or flight" hormones don't dissipate. Once the immediate alarm passes, your hormones orchestrate physical and psychological coping. One common response is a signal to eat. If you

"I own a business, so I'm in charge of everyone," Tom said. *"But I'm also where the buck stops on all the problems—a million things go wrong in construction, and my guys have constant personal problems I hear about, too. Yeah, I've got stress. A beer and the news at the end of the day are how I 'come down' from my crazy day. I know I could be healthier but, man, the TV and beer works."*

don't find ways to control your stress, "fight or flight" can turn into what stress researcher Pamela Peeke, MD, calls "stew and chew."

One stress hormone in particular, called cortisone, can trigger overeating and make our bodies collect what Dr. Peeke, in her excellent book *Fight Fat After Forty*, calls "toxic fat," the deadly result of eating too much of the wrong foods at the wrong times. Dr. Peeke describes the "cortizone" (a word-play on the hormone cortisone) as the period late in the day when, for many women, stress-related, high-fat, high-starch eating occurs. Overeating during the evening "cortizone" tends to be more difficult to control, and the resulting fat tends to accumulate in the belly. More of this abdominal "toxic fat" is associated with a medical problem called "metabolic syndrome," a deadly combo of high blood pressure, high blood lipid levels, high insulin levels, and insulin resistance. And, as a woman enters menopause and her hormone profile changes, her likelihood of accumulating this toxic fat increases. So, stress management with movement such as yoga not only makes you feel good, it can save your life.

The female factor

Until shockingly recently, medical science was based only on men's bodies. The complex and powerful female hormonal system was completely ignored. As women are included in medical studies, the differences in response to treatments and drugs pile up. We now know that a woman's hormonal system, and specifically estrogen, makes fat cells more likely to form and less likely to break down. Estrogen also determines where fat accumulates—in the breasts, abdomen, and hips.

"That's definitely me," said Barbara. "I've noticed that my weight just stopped bouncing back when I'd been on an overeating jag and tried to be better for a few days. The extra pound or two just stayed put."

"I see it too," said Suzanne. "There's a permanence or thickness to my belly that was just never part of my body until the past few years. At least now I know what's happening."

Again, heredity collides with modern life to backfire on our weight-loss schemes. Men have the body composition and therefore the metabolic advantage too. Men have an average 12% body fat to women's 20%. So, if you have ever tried to lose weight in partnership with a man, and watched his pounds melt off while yours didn't, you have seen his larger muscle mass and fat-burning hormonal environment at work.

As you age, your body tends to lose muscle and bone, and to gain fat. Fat doesn't use calories as muscle does. Starting around age 40, women can lose about one-third of a pound of muscle and some bone each year, with an accompanying downshift in metabolism. The good news, again, is that much of this loss, both muscle and bone, can be prevented through conscious eating and becoming and remaining physically active.

What Is a Healthy Weight Lifestyle?

The truth (and the reason for the national confusion) is that there are many, many paths to good health and to healthy eating. As you build the lifestyle that works for you, remember there are many sources of sound guidance. I've listed my favorites in the Resources for Further Study section of this book. There are a few universal truths, however, that, regardless of your personal choices of how and what to eat, bear up well under the light of scientific scrutiny. Despite what you hear in the media, the basics of a healthy lifestyle haven't changed in the last 50 years. There is lots of debate, however, about the details.

Following are some basic time-tested principles:

1) **A healthy lifestyle is one that you can stick to without feeling deprived.** Be it vegetarian, the Zone, Atkins, Weight Watchers, Eat Right 4 Your Type, or most other plans out there, a healthy lifestyle is one that nourishes your body without messing with your mind. You can stick with it for the rest of your life, not just for a month or two while you're losing weight. Some diets have a more restrictive "cleansing phase," which can be fine if you know it won't backfire. If you know you are a compulsive eater or binger, deprivation has a funny way of backfiring into a diet-binge cycle. Likewise, doing exercises you hate won't last long, and you probably won't give it your all, so you may even burn fewer calories doing it.

2) **A healthy diet relies on plants: fruits, vegetables, and whole grains.** The science is clear. Meat and animal products can be part of a healthy diet, but whole grains and plenty of fruits and vegetables provide the fiber and nutrients in such short supply in our fast-food, over-processed culture. Aim for at least five servings of fruit and/or vegetables every single day. The optimal number is nine to ten daily servings.

3) **A healthy diet nourishes your body: it has enough calories to meet your basic metabolic needs.** Starvation diets don't work (and are no fun at all!). The deprivation mindset they engender can have an impact on your entire life. You can't lose weight permanently without feeding your body and having the energy to be physically active. Wouldn't it be great to not be in the deprivation mindset ever again? Actually, it's the only way.

4) **A healthy lifestyle is a physically active lifestyle.** The interplay of eating and movement is an ever-evolving dance. You just can't be active unless you eat. Becoming active often makes people more interested in eating a healthy, balanced diet. No matter who you are—how old, what color, what neighborhood, or your physical condition—being active can change your life for the better.

5) **A healthy lifestyle is individualized: it reflects your age, health history, social and financial needs, preferences, and temperament.** Your best diet is as individual as you are. It takes into account the food you like to eat and whether you like to cook or are a take-out connoisseur. It's one you can afford without taking a second job. Your stage of life, gender, and the diseases that run in your family all play a role in what's on your plate.

6) **A healthy diet is fat-savvy.** Diets high in animal and processed fats lead, over time, to a myriad of health problems. The shift from artery-clogging saturated and trans fats to healthier vegetable and fish oils can make you feel better and live longer.

7) **A healthy diet is moderate and varied.** Moderation. We all know it's important, but do we really know what moderation is? In our anything-but-moderate culture, there are few examples to follow. That's where yoga comes in. The moderate yogi is no passive snoozer, but a strong and practiced warrior standing in the fire between overindulgence and deprivation. The exercises in this book will help you learn to listen to your body and your emotions to recognize when you veer out of your moderate zone.

No one recipe, even if followed to a tee, will deliver a healthy diet to absolutely everyone. The guidelines above are flexible truths that can guide your exploration toward your healthiest diet. The important thing is to stay on your path, revel in the fullness of your humanity (your strengths and your limitations), and live your fullest, most soul-filled life. Your journey won't happen overnight, or over a weekend, or even in 30 days. It will take the rest of your life. The good news is that you are already on your way by exploring the ideas in this book.

Eastern contemplative philosophies such as yoga can provide a life framework for making the shifts of perception necessary to adopt a healthier lifestyle. Chapter Two, on yoga and meditation, gives you an introduction to that process and its underlying rationale.

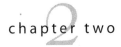
yoga and meditation: an alchemy of awareness

In order to live in this duplicitous consumer culture, we often go numb rather than be fully aware of just how destructive to our bodies and our souls popular culture really can be.

To lead healthy lives we somehow need to find the ability to pull away from the glow of the tube and reconnect with our real physical, emotional, intellectual, and spiritual needs. Here is where yoga, a practice developed over five thousand years ago, seems a gift perfect for us today.

— KRIPALU TEACHER TRAINING MANUAL

What Is Yoga?

Let's begin at the beginning. Yoga is an ancient philosophical system originating in India whose beginnings may be traced as far back as 5,000 BCE. The word *yoga* comes from the Sanskrit root *yuj*, which means "to bind, join, attach, and yoke," or "to use and apply." It also means "union" or "communion." Sanskrit* is an ancient language no longer commonly spoken except within spiritual or educational situations. It is the language in which yoga was developed. Sanskrit is a beautifully lyrical language, and its use in yoga practice gives us a sensory link to its history. While yoga in America today often focuses only on the physical practice (asana), the full practice of yoga encompasses every aspect of life, including diet, mental attitude, and choices about lifestyle and philosophical study.

The Bhagavad-Gita is the earliest surviving text that just focuses solely on yoga. It is a self-contained portion of a Hindu epic, the Mahabharata, written at about 450 BCE. The Bhagavad-Gita is a fable that recounts the dialogue between the disillusioned warrior prince Arjuna and Lord Krishna. Krishna is an incarnation of Vishnu, the second deity of the Hindu trinity, entrusted with the preservation of the world. The Bhagavad-Gita teaches the way of renunciation in action as a means of navigating a seemingly impossible situation: Arjuna may fight a just war between two sides of his own family as long as he is able to control his senses and actions without desire or ego. He must learn to step back from the heat of his emotional attachments and aversions, and act from abiding calm. According to scholar Chip Hartranft, in this text Krishna teaches Arjuna about two dimensions of human awareness: that our true nature is hidden but abides in pure awareness when the veil of physical being is drawn aside, and that transcendent love empowers the seeker to relate personally to the divine.

Another early Eastern philosopher with a complimentary take on the process of internal focusing is Siddhartha Gautama (the Buddha), who lived from about 563-483 BCE. He proposed that liberation occurs

---

* Sanskrit is a complex and ancient language. Many of the Sanskrit words included in this text contain various diacritics (accent marks) in their most correct forms. For English readability, and because various yoga texts differ on diacritics for a given term, they have been eliminated in this book.

"So the Bhagavad-Gita is about becoming more aware of how you can shift the way that you see things, right?" asked Suzanne. "Yes," I replied. "It describes the process of yoga, the process of consciously shifting your perspective, and it suggests that the transcendence we sometimes feel can deepen more than we can imagine." "You know, I can see in my life how stepping back and taking a breath helps me make better decisions," Suzanne noted. "But the idea that my yoga practice will help me to do that, and at the same time prepare me to experience more peace or transcendence…that's pretty motivating, and I like that thread between the ancient yogis and my life today."

when things are seen as they actually are. He said when consciousness is no longer constrained by wanting or aversion, awareness opens to the unconditioned, or nirvana (literally, "extinguished"). The Buddha proposed an "eightfold path" to freedom, which may have influenced the sage Patanjali's later "eight-limbed path" of yoga, the Yoga Sutra.

The Philosophy of Yoga

> *The posture of yoga is steady and easy.*
> *It is realized by relaxing one's effort and resting like*
> *the cosmic serpent on the waters of infinity.*
> *Then one is unconstrained by opposing dualities.*

—YOGA SUTRA OF PATANJALI II:46-48

The Yoga Sutra, written by Patanjali in approximately 250 CE describes the practice and philosophy of yoga in 196 brief sutras, or phrase-threads. An essential guide for studying yoga and Eastern spirituality, the Yoga Sutra is recognized for both its sophistication and its poetic simplicity. In it, Patanjali describes the nature of human suffering, and then describes a meditation-based plan for living through which the practitioner can fulfill the primary purpose of consciousness: to see things as they are, thus achieving freedom from suffering.

Patanjali's eight-limbed path of yoga includes:

1) **Yamas:** controls or restraints of attitude or behavior, primarily in community or relationship. These include:

   Ahimsa: non-violence, compassion

   Satya: truthfulness

   Asteya: non-stealing

   Brahmacharya: chastity or control of the life force

   Aparigraha: greedlessness or charity

2) **Niyamas:** observances and attitudes primarily concerned with the individual. These include:

   Saucha: purity, cleanliness

   Santosa: contentment

   Tapas: asceticism, simplicity, passion

   Svadhyaya: self-study, self-inquiry, philosophical study

   Isvara Pranidhana: devotion to God

The remaining limbs of yoga according to Patanjali are:

3) **Asana:** literally means "seat" and describes the physical practice of yoga postures.

4) **Pranayama:** controlling energy and breath.

5) **Pratyahara:** inward focusing and withdrawal of the senses.

6) **Dharana:** focused concentration.

7) **Dhyana:** meditation.

8) **Samadhi:** absorption into bliss consciousness.

The first two limbs of yoga provide the framework for what yogis refer to as "right livelihood"—living in such a way as to decrease suffering, both individually and universally. The yamas and niyamas describe how a conscious, realized human acts. As a yogi (male practitioner of yoga) or yogini (female practitioner) moves along this path, the meaning of the yamas and niyamas are likely to deepen. One model describing how this deepening may proceed, explored by the Kripalu Center for Health and others, is shown in Chart 5. Yoga is an experiential practice, so the meaning of the practice will unfold in as many ways as there are individuals; the layers described here are just one possibility.

Yoga Psychology

Everyone wants to be happy. But we all know how elusive happiness often is, even for the most intelligent and best intentioned. Nearly everyone, however, has had moments of transcendence or deep connection. The swell of emotion on the first glimpse of your child being born or being overwhelmed by an expansive star-filled sky brings lucid focus to the present moment. Yoga, meditation, and other contemplative practices are tools for cultivating the ability to dwell in the present moment and to have more awareness of the transcendent possibility of every moment of our lives.

From a spiritual perspective, contemplative practices facilitate the process of joining individual consciousness with universal consciousness. According to Kripalu scholar Stephen Cope, the Sanskrit word *Samkya* describes the underlying dualistic worldview that holds that spirit (purusha) and matter (prakrti) appear to be separate. That is, the aspect of our being sometimes referred to as "the witness" or our knowing presence is distinct and different from the natural world that encompasses our physical body, our conscious reality, and all that we

Chart 5: Yamas and Niyamas

Yama/ Niyama	Layer One	Layer Two	Layer Three	Layer Four	Layer Five	Layer Six
Non-violence (ahimsa)	No physical injury or verbal abuse to others	No physical or verbal abuse to yourself	No negative deeds	No negative thoughts	Loving service	Being universal love
Truthfulness (satya)	No lies in speech	No pretense, no lies to yourself	No opinions	Speak seldom and carefully	Silent—too hard to speak truth	Being universal truth
Non-stealing (asteya)	Not taking what isn't yours, cultivating integrity	Not trying to get more than you need	Not wanting more than you need	Not accepting more than you need	Not wanting anything	Being everything
Non-possessiveness (aparigraha)	No greed, cultivating generosity	Reducing wants and needs	Letting go of what you don't need	Freedom from opinions	Living in non-judgmental consciousness	Being it all
Personal energy management (brahmacharya)	Moderation in all sense pleasures, celibacy outside marriage	No compulsion to seek sense pleasures	No wish to seek sense pleasures	Free from dualistic thinking	Constant awareness of inner joy	Unceasing inner ecstasy replaces outward focus
Purification (saucha)	Physical: clean pure diet, yoga postures, physical activity	Emotional: riding the wave, pranayama	Mental: good company, high thinking, meditation	Intellect: Discriminate rather than reactive	Established in bliss body	Being pure energy, able to take form as you wish
Contentment (santosa)	Enjoyment of and gratitude for all you have	Gratitude for even the unpleasant experience	Contentment independent of what the mind thinks	"The Great Way is easy for those who have no preferences."	Predispositions and cultural conditioning neutralized.	Being the Self, content in the Self
Transformation (tapas)	Simplify, self-discipline, follow through on your intentions	Observance of self-chosen vows, fasts, and austerities	Experiencing all feelings without resistance	Receiving all life experience without resistance	Mastery of physical, mental, and spiritual bodies	Self-creative, consciousness
Self-study (svadhyaya)	Spiritual study and investigation	Objective non-judgmental self-observation	Noticing and imbibing inspiring qualities of others	Living in balance with your life energy: prana	Living from and directed by universal prana	Being the universal energy: prana
Surrender to the Universal Divinity (Isvara pranidhana)	Desire to serve	Selfless service outside your family	A life of service as an instrument of universal divinity	Each action fulfills self, others, and is grounded	Being an instrument of universal divinity	Being divine without division

Source: Kripalu Center for Yoga and Health. Adapted from the Kripalu Teacher Training Manual, 2006.

see around us. According to these teachings, our awareness interacts with the natural world through the physical body. Unfortunately, in the process of this interaction, awareness forgets that it is unlimited, boundless, and divine, and begins to see itself as bound, separate from the universe, and restricted. Like Buddhism and other Eastern practices, yoga turns attention inward so that ultimately our awareness can remember itself as unlimited. This turning inward of attention and self-observation with an attitude of compassion described in the Yoga Sutras lies at the heart of yoga psychology.

As you gain skill as a yoga practitioner, your sense of physical, psychological, and emotional realities often shift, becoming less influenced by the external forces of modern culture and more anchored in your internal value system. You more easily recognize your own divinity. This is the cognitive restructuring within the practice of yoga that makes it a valuable tool for supporting health behavior change. By using physical sensation within one's own body as a focal point, yoga personalizes the context of our actions, and of our change. We learn to relate bodily physical sensations to emotions and gain skill in differentiating sensations and their physical, emotional, and energetic messages.

What Is Meditation?

Meditation is a process of quieting the physical body and the mind. Yoga scholar Georg Feurerstein, PhD, describes meditative absorption (dhyana) as the state of deep concentration in which the internalized object fills the entire space of consciousness. All arising ideas, notes Feurerstein, gyrate around the object of concentration and are accompanied by a peaceful mental disposition. There is no loss of lucidity, but the sense of wakefulness appears to be intensified even though there is little awareness of the external environment.

There are a number of theories investigating the physiology of how yoga, meditation, and other mind-body modalities work. One is that yoga practice helps to fine-tune our sensory systems, which have internal, external, and memory components. On a conscious level we can normally be aware of only one of these three components. In yoga and other contemplative practices, however, we practice the interplay of these components and begin to develop the ability to be simultaneously aware of our internal, external, and memory realities, thus gaining insight into how events in our lives imprint our sensory system and therefore our bodies.

Meditation is increasingly recognized as having clinical effects. These include a broad spectrum of physical benefits, such as reduced anxiety, pain, depression, and stress, along with enhanced mood and self-esteem. Meditation is a hot area of research and has been studied in people with fibromyalgia, cancer, hypertension, carpal tunnel syndrome, and psoriasis. Both the quality and the quantity of research in this area are growing. In a study by Davidson and Kabat-Zinn, a short program in mindfulness meditation produced demonstrable improvements in brain and immune function.

How Yoga and Meditation Aid Weight Management

As we've seen, living in the American culture and maintaining a healthy weight can seem mutually exclusive. Let's now look at how yoga and meditation can help.

The practices of yoga, breath-based stress management, and meditation, with their elements of clarifying internal vs. external values, development of the skills to differentiate between reality and delusion, and provision of physical context for emotional work, provide useful tools for these challenging personal transitions. As you develop your practice and become more familiar with your internal cues, you may become less influenced by the external values of beauty and excessive thinness projected in the media.

After a few yoga sessions, Barbara came to me and said, "Exercising for an hour every day, the way the health groups say I should, is just not going to happen right now. It would be great, sure. But sometimes I feel like I can barely make it up the stairs to my house. But these yoga classes are gentle enough that I can hang in there for an hour class—it's a little less daunting. No performance, spandex, or strain." Suzanne, standing nearby, added, "There's something about knowing that I am combining physical activity with stress management that really appeals to the multitasking part of me! And, I can adjust the difficulty level up or down, so like Barbara, I'm relieved it's really accessible."

Traditional weight management therapy in combination with yoga and meditation practice may be particularly well suited to interested women whose weight accumulates in their bellies. As discussed, belly fat in women may be a response to chronic stress, and it increases risk for a number of chronic health conditions. Yoga can provide gentle physical activity and the cognitive shifting that can support the adoption of healthy behaviors, all the while providing stress management.

In addition to its stress management benefits, yoga, and particularly the yamas and niyamas, is helpful in defining moderation. Many national health organizations feature moderation in their guidelines, but are light on the how-to's of achieving a moderate lifestyle in our anything-but-moderate culture. In the yoga philosophy moderation is not a passive state, but is more akin to "standing in the fire" between the two beckoning poles of excess and deprivation. The moderate yogini is no passive risk-avoider, but is a highly skilled and strong-willed warrior. The practice of yoga and meditation may assist the development of mindfulness during mealtimes, aiding awareness of portion sizes, food preparation, and eating speed.

Yoga is a vehicle for training your mind to think clearly, calmly, and kindly. That journey of exploring your mind's ways occurs within your physical body. Learning to hear and interpret your body's messages can help you recognize and discern the physical sensations of emotion, stress, and disease. This ability to reconnect to sensation is in essence the mind-body connection. It can profoundly change your life. And it's the reason why coupling nutrition with yoga is an excellent way to adopt a healthier lifestyle.

Yoga and meditation may not be useful in all situations of weight management. For those interested, however, these practices can offer a mental paradigm shift and the gentle physical activity that may uniquely support healthy attitudes about weight, eating, and self-care. Chapter Three: Self-Discovery: Exploring Lifestyle Choices will help you begin your journey.

chapter three

self-discovery:
exploring lifestyle choices

It is helpful to realize that this very body that we have,
sitting right here right now…with its aches and its pleasures…
is exactly what we need to be fully human, fully awake, fully alive.

— PEMA CHÖDRÖN

The following five chapters outline a process of using yoga philosophy and practice to enhance your awareness of your physical body, mental landscape, and lifestyle habits. Then, you can slowly adjust those habits and their underlying mental frameworks in order to enhance your health and well-being. Your journey toward wholeness can be aided at any time by an experienced yoga teacher and a nutrition professional, the best of whose life work is facilitating people like you on their way.

Beginning with this chapter, it will be helpful to use a journal for written exercises and for your own exploration. Keeping your thoughts and insights on paper will motivate you and give you a record of your progress. Your journal notes will remind you of what works for you and what doesn't.

Setting Intention

"Intention is the thread that forms a necklace on which the pearls of life experience are strung."

— KRIPALU TEACHER MARCIA GOLDBERG (SHANTIPRIYA)

Why do you want to lose weight? And what is your ideal weight? The vast majority of mature people set an ideal weight for themselves that they have not seen since junior high school. It may be possible to reach that weight if their entire life is dedicated to the feat. But, they likely would not recognize nor choose that life. Nevertheless, many hold that ideal as their goal, suffering in self-imposed failure even before they begin. Barbara was no exception.

Unrealistic goals are a natural fallout from our delusion-promoting culture that tells us that everyone is thin, happy, young, and rich, and that to be otherwise (which we all, eventually, are) is abject failure. But in fact, if you are overweight, just losing 10% of your body weight can result in significant improvements in health. And, there is a growing body of science that suggests that it is our habits more than the number on the scale that determines our overall weight-health. Can you see how much needless suffering is wrapped up setting unrealistic goals? The sooner we can release expectations and begin a process of paying attention to the here and now, the happier we will be. And we'll take better care of ourselves.

One of the first questions I asked Barbara and others in the workshop was:
"What is your ideal weight?"
"I want to weigh 130. I felt so good at that weight," she said.
"When was the last time you weighed 130?" I asked.
"Oh gosh, it must have been in college, over 20 years ago…"

Intention flowers from our core values. Values define who we are and what is important to us. If we live without intention, we tend to be easily swayed by the latest fad and quickly redirected away from the things that are most important to us. So, our lives will likely have a haphazard or superficial quality. By cultivating intention, we greatly enhance the likelihood that what we most value will guide our lives.

Here is an exercise drawn from Marcia Goldberg's work to help you explore your intentions around self-care.

After the intention exercise, I asked Barbara again, "Why do you want to lose weight?" The exercise allowed her to go deeper. "I want to lead a fuller, happier life," she said. "I want to feel better about myself, and more connected with who I am."

Exercise 1: Intention

1) In your journal, write down, in your own words, an intention to deeply nurture yourself. Then, come into a position on the floor that feels nurturing. Stay there until you begin to feel the urge to move. Notice if this urge comes from your thinking mind or a physical sensation in the body. Wait for the physical sensations that signal your body's desire to adjust. Then let your body move and adjust to deepen the experience of nurturance. Open to receive nurturance from this new position. Continuing with the intention of self-nurturance, spend the next 15 minutes listening and responding to the messages of your body. Notice any thoughts in your mind, and simply watch them as a compassionate observer. Once you become familiar with the experience of setting an intention and letting the actions come from the signals of prana (life force) responding to the request, it becomes easier to apply this to daily life.

2) Identify a quality that you would like to develop in your life. Go outside, finding a place where you can comfortably be quiet and still. Take several relaxed breaths. Relax and connect with the earth, sky, or whatever is around you. You may want to walk slowly or be still. See if you can let yourself be guided by inner sensation. Carry your intention with you, seeking its presence

through connection to the elements of nature. Then take your intention into your life by opening yourself up to finding it in daily activities. For example, imagine that your intention is abundance. "I feel the abundance of sunlight on my skin and the sounds around me as I sit on the hillside. I notice that the field holds abundant blades of grass. The breeze stirs the trees and wind chimes, creating nuances of sound I have never noticed before. There is more than enough air to breathe. It fills my lungs fully. The colors around me are abundant—shades of brown and green of early spring. This moment is an eternity—abundant time."

Your Weight Reality Project: Self-Assessment

"I hate scales," was the first thing Barbara said to me as the discussion began. "Please don't make me weigh myself." Was I surprised? No. For those of us who struggle with weight and eating, getting on that small bathroom appliance can feel like stepping onto the great scales of judgment.

When it comes to your personal weight story, the number on the scale is only the beginning. But the first step in any journey is figuring out where you are and getting a clear idea of your destination. That's where self-assessment comes in. Here you will note a few simple measures that can help you determine just what your weight reality is. Gathering this information will help to map the most productive course for your efforts on finding your natural weight.

Body Mass Index (BMI)

For some of us, gathering numbers and taking measurements is enough to make us close this book, make a nice big bowl of buttered popcorn and burrow in for a *Law and Order* marathon. If you have a similar reaction, you are having the perfectly normal experience of your mind resisting your reality project. Part of your mind would love things to stay the same; it likes popcorn and *Law and Order*! And,

Chart 6: Body Mass Index (BMI)

$$BMI = \left\{ \frac{WEIGHT\ (pounds)}{HEIGHT\ (inches)^2} \right\} \times 703$$

Weight in Pounds

Height in Feet and Inches	120	130	140	150	160	170	180	190	200	210	220	230	240	250
4'6"	29	31	34	36	39	41	43	46	48	51	53	56	58	60
4'8"	27	29	31	34	36	38	40	43	45	47	49	52	54	56
4'10"	25	27	29	31	34	36	38	40	42	44	46	48	50	52
5'0"	23	25	27	29	31	33	35	37	39	41	43	45	47	49
5'2"	22	24	26	27	29	31	33	35	37	38	40	42	44	46
5'4"	21	22	24	26	28	29	31	33	34	36	38	40	41	43
5'6"	19	21	23	24	26	27	29	31	32	34	36	37	39	40
5'8"	18	20	21	23	24	26	27	29	30	32	34	35	37	38
5'10"	17	19	20	22	23	24	26	27	29	30	32	33	35	36
6'0"	16	18	19	20	22	23	24	26	27	28	30	31	33	34
6'2"	15	17	18	19	21	22	23	24	26	27	28	30	31	32
6'4"	15	16	17	18	20	21	22	23	24	26	27	28	29	30
6'6"	14	15	16	17	19	20	21	22	23	24	25	27	28	29
6'8"	13	14	15	17	18	19	20	21	22	23	24	25	26	28

Healthy Weight　　Overweight　　Obese

Note: *This chart is for adults (aged 20 years and older).*

Source: Centers for Disease Control (CDC)

there are real benefits to the habits that cause us to be overweight; they are familiar and comforting. But once you realize what your mind is trying to do, the gig is pretty much up. Sorry, you're conscious! Waking up to the mind's evasive maneuvering to avoid change has a funny way of taking the pleasure out of burying your head in the sand of TV and snacking.

Your Body Mass Index (BMI) is an estimate of your weight status and indirectly your body fat, based on your height and weight. Once you measure your weight and height you can find your BMI on a

"OK," said Barbara. "I'm feeling the resistance but doing it anyway. My weight is 240 pounds, and my height is 5'8", so my BMI is 37. OK, I'm in the obese category, but it does feel good to face it. This is where I start." "Keep in mind," I added, "that your BMI is just one estimate and doesn't directly reflect your level of fitness. Someone may be healthier at a higher BMI if they are active and eat well than someone with a lower BMI but poor habits." "Oh," said Barbara. "So you're saying even though I'm obese, I can get healthier right away by taking better care of myself." "Beautiful!"

chart like Chart 6, through a growing number of Internet sites (some are listed in the Resources for Further Study section of this book), or you can calculate it yourself from the BMI equation, in Chart 6.

Waist measurement

Next, measure your waist. Why? Because excess abdominal fat is an independent predictor of health problems. Increased risk for weight-related problems occurs with waist circumference of more than 40 inches in men and more than 35 inches in women. Having a high waist circumference is associated with diabetes, high cholesterol, high blood pressure, and heart disease for people with a BMI between 25 to just shy of 35. The waist circumference is less predictive for people with a BMI of 35 or over. Note your BMI and waist circumference in your journal.

"Measuring my waist was another chance to overcome resistance…I'm getting better at it," said Barbara. "My waist is 39 inches, so while my BMI puts me in a place where high waist circumference is less predictive, for me it's just one more sign that, yes, I need to do something about this."

Your Health Barriers and Resources

Now that you have collected some of the basic measures of your weight reality—your weight, your BMI, and your waist circumference—

46

Chart 7: Measuring Tape Position for Waist (Abdominal) Circumference

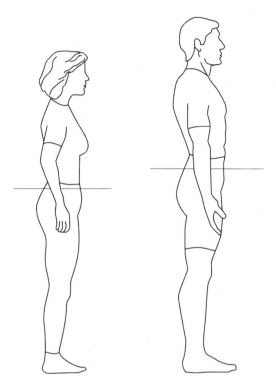

you can complete your self-assessment by considering your risk and resource profile. Your risk and resource profile influences your chances of experiencing weight-related health complications. The equation for anticipating your risk of illness is complex and would take the remainder of this book to describe and assess in detail. So for the sake of your weight reality project, just know that the more factors listed in Chart 8 that apply to you, the greater your likelihood that being overweight is not just a cosmetic inconvenience, but may have some real health fallout. Note your risk factors in your journal. Remember, the good news is that you can change much of your risk profile by changing your lifestyle. Can you see these factors as messages and motivators rather than fatal flaws?

Chart 8: Factors That Increase Health Risks for People of Size

Disease conditions	• Coronary heart disease or other atherosclerotic disease • Type 2 diabetes • Sleep apnea
Other obesity-associated diseases	• Gynecological problems • Osteoarthritis • Gallstones • Stress incontinence
Cardiovascular risk factors	• Cigarette smoking • High blood pressure (systolic $\geq$ 140 mmHg or diastolic $\geq$ 90 mmHg), or antihypertensive medication • High-risk LDL cholesterol ($\geq$ 160 mg/dL) • Low HDL cholesterol (< 35 mg/dL) • Impaired fasting glucose (fasting plasma glucose of 110-125 mg/dL) • Family history of heart attack at or before 55 years of age in father or other male first-degree relative, or at or before 65 years of age in mother or other female first-degree relative • Age $\geq$ 45 years (men) • $\geq$ 55 years (women)
Other risk factors	• Physical inactivity • High serum triglycerides (> 200 mg/dL)

Source: National Institute of Health. *Clinical Guidelines of the Identification, Evaluation, and Treatment of Overweight and Obesity in Adults. The Evidence Report.* NIH Publication no. 98-4083. Sept 1998.

"I have a number of the cardiovascular risk factors," notes Barbara. "So I'll lean toward a heart-healthy lifestyle and make an effort to learn more about what that means. I am finding, as I get support from this group, that I can build my life resources in the right direction. I've always had a problem with being motivated, but with this support I'm getting better. My mental attitude is definitely improving even though I now see in black and white that my weight is a real health issue. I feel ready to make some changes."

When a nutrition professional explores your motivation to make lifestyle change, she will ask you about a number of things that provide clues as to how big your challenge of change may be. Chart 9 lists just some of the resources in your life that may support your ability to change your habits. Can you think of more?

Chart 9: Life Resources That Support Successful Habit Change

- **Healthy motivators.** Reasons for pursuing weight loss independent of physical appearance or external value systems such as the media or peer desires. Examples of supportive reasons may include to become healthier, to feel better, and to get stronger.

- **A track record.** Previous history of successful behavior change. If you have quit smoking or adopted other positive habits, you have an understanding of the process of change, which may support your effort. If your weight has "cycled" (i.e., you have repeatedly gained and lost weight), that may be either a barrier or a supporter, depending upon what you have learned.

- **Support.** Positive friends, family, and worksites make following a healthy lifestyle much easier.

- **Accurate knowledge.** An understanding of the medical consequences of weight may motivate you. The ability to separate fact from fad in the sea of dietary misinformation will save you lots of time.

- **Attitude.** A positive attitude toward the idea that adopting a healthy lifestyle can be fun and pleasurable.

Lifestyle Manifestation

Everything you have been doing so far has been about starting to explore a lifestyle that is right for you. Now you are ready for an exercise to help you begin to map your own steps to successful lifestyle manifestation. Use your journal to record your responses.

Reframing the struggle

The life resources you found in Chart 9 are gems that you can look to when things get tough. And, as for the aspects of your life that may feel like obstacles to wellness now, well, counter-intuitive as it may seem, it is the aspects of our lives that feel like barriers to being whom or what we want to be that can hold our greatest gifts. For those of us who struggle with weight and eating, just imagine the ocean of compassion we need to summon in order to consider that struggle our gift! And how much courage must be summoned to then dive into the struggle and hold it up to the light.

Yoga and other Eastern philosophies suggest that if we have the courage to explore our deepest pain with clear-eyed compassion, we may very well find the answer to our deepest longing. The process of making the journey is no less than our personal path to physical, mental, and spiritual nourishment. Let the possibility of hearing the quiet voice within you compel you to take the next step. Remember, too, that tens of thousands of yogis for thousands of years have told us that what we will find when we make this journey to the center of our being is not a ball of terror or a black hole, but something very, very good—the light of our own divinity.

Exercise 2: Steps to Successful Lifestyle Manifestation

The purpose of this exercise is to help you begin and maintain the journey toward conscious, healthful eating habits by exploring your existing habits. The steps outlined below will guide you in (1) identifying your intention in changing, (2) identifying habits or areas for improvement, (3) using affirmations and setting realistic and achievable goals, and (4) developing an achievable plan of action and a system for learning from inevitable setbacks.

1) **Set an intention.** An intention may be inspired by the yamas and niyamas of yoga philosophy (outlined in Chapter Two).

   What is your intention for this process? What are you interested in bringing in or developing? What is your body, your mind, your soul seeking through this experience?

2) **Identify areas for improvement.** Use information from your most recent self-monitoring and/or past experience to identify areas for dietary improvement. List the three areas that are most important to you.

   1.

   2.

   3.

3) **Set a goal.** Select one area for improvement from the list you made above. Your goal must be specific, measurable, and realistic. Answer all the questions that apply to the area that you have selected for modification.

   What is your area to modify?

   What will you do differently so that you know (or someone else observing you knows) that you are making progress toward your goal?

   Specify a time period (e.g., week, month, vacation)

   Specify how often (e.g., daily, once a week)

   Specify how much (e.g., ½ cup, 1 oz., 30 min.)

   Specify where (e.g., home, restaurant, work)

   Specify with whom (e.g., family member, friends, co-workers)

4) **Develop affirmations.** These are clear statements of what you want to create, which can support your goal. They are the fruit of your intention, and they bring intention deeper into your daily being.

Affirmations are:

⌐ Written down

⌐ Succinct

⌐ Specific

⌐ Stated in the present tense

⌐ Stated in the positive

⌐ Strongly evocative for you personally

⌐ Addressed to yourself (and include you); not about changing others

What are some affirmations that may support your goal?

5) **Visualize your goal.** The mental images we most frequently hold are what we manifest. Visualization will:

⌐ Give you a strong positive feeling when you hold it

⌐ Include you in the picture, doing your vision with fulfillment

⌐ Be either literal or metaphoric

⌐ Be written down and/or drawn as a picture

Visualize yourself practicing a behavior that will help you reach your goal. Write or draw your supportive visualization.

6) **Develop a plan of action.** List the three challenges that you are most likely to encounter in your effort to reach your goal.

Challenge #1:

Challenge #2:

Challenge #3:

What will you do to manage your challenges in order to prevent them from affecting your ability to attain your goal?

To manage challenge #1, I will:

To manage challenge #2, I will:

To manage challenge #3, I will:

7) **Explore achievability.** How confident are you, on a scale of 0-100%, that you can achieve this goal?

0%   10%   20%   30%   40%   50%   60%   70%   80%   90%   100%

(If you are not at least 75% confident, modify your goal to increase the likelihood that you will be successful.)

8) **Embody your intention.** Live now what you intend to manifest. You create what you confidently expect to create. To germinate the mental seed, create a feeling of expectation and assumption that it is already manifesting for you, in you. What supports this feeling of certainty is:

A) Daily repetition: as often as you can remember to

B) Walking your talk: move, speak, and carry yourself as one who is this vision and has already achieved it

C) Ongoing clearing: of the self to keep your thoughts supportive of the vision

D) Alignment with inner attunement: your higher purpose for existing as a spiritual/human being

9) **Seal the deal with a contract.** Write up an iron-clad agreement with yourself. Here is one example:

I will begin working on the following goal and supporting affirmations:
On (date), I will self-monitor or journal to evaluate my success in reaching my goal, (your goal), and discuss successes and challenges with (who you'll check in with) on (date).

(Sign and date your goal, and make any additional notes.)

Here is how Barbara responded to this exercise:

1) **Set an intention.**

   What is your intention for this process? What are you interested in bringing in or developing? What is your body, your mind, your soul seeking through this experience?

   I want to lead a full and happy life—I want to feel better about myself and feel more connected with who I am.

2) **Identify areas for improvement.** List the three areas that are most important to you.

   1. *overeating, especially at night*

   2. *not exercising regularly*

   3. *beating up on myself—something with my frame of mind*

3) **Set a goal.**

   Area to modify: *not exercising enough*

   What will you do differently so that you know (or someone else observing you knows) that you are making progress toward your goal? *I will either work in the garden, take an exercise class, or walk for at least 30 minutes most (5) days (or do some other exercise), and I will start a meditation practice of 5 minutes/day at least 5 days each week.*

   Specify a time period (e.g., week, month, vacation):
   over the next month

   Specify how often (e.g., daily, once a week): *5x/week*

   Specify how much (e.g., ½ cup, 1 oz., 30 min.):
   30 minutes minimum activity, 5 minutes meditation

   Specify where (e.g., home, restaurant, work):
   home or club or yoga

   Specify with whom (e.g., family member, friends, co-workers):
   alone or with a friend

4) Affirmations to support my goal:

I love movement. I can have fun being active.

I believe activity is part of a whole and happy life.

I have control over my day and my schedule.

I believe that being active and being still are essential components of who I am.

5) Visualize your goal.

There I am—beautiful Barbara at my best, a mature, strong, and quietly confident woman with a full life that does not overwhelm me. Grace under pressure. It's a dark and rainy day, the kids have gotten off to school, and after taking a few minutes to quiet down, I pop in a yoga CD. Just as I settle in, the phone rings—I don't get up, but listen to the message—it's my husband, who wonders if I would like to go to the Clam Shak for an early lunch with my favorite co-worker of his. I don't get up—I will complete my work here for 30 minutes and then call him back. They will either still be there or not. I relax. I breathe. And begin my work.

6) Develop a plan of action.

Challenge #1: *energy level/motivation*

Challenge #2: *planning/schedule/commitments—distractions!*

Challenge #3: *husband offering non-active alternatives for free time!*

To manage challenge #1, I will:

1. Find activities where I can still move a bit, even when I don't feel like it.

2. Know the classes I like that I can go to on low-motivation days.

3. Find and stay in touch with others trying to be healthy.

4. Just do it—feel the emotion (unmotivated, tired) and be active anyway, but in a way that honors my emotion (if I can do that, I don't know)

To manage challenge #2, I will:

Plan exercise into every day. Be aware of the best time to exercise—when I'll actually follow through.

To manage challenge #3, I will:

Talk to my husband about these goals and ask for his support.

7) **Explore achievability.** How confident are you, on a scale of 0-100%, that you can achieve this goal?

0%   10%   20%   30%   40%   (50%)   60%   70%   80%   90%   100%

(If you are not at least 75% confident, modify your goal to increase the likelihood that you will be successful.)

If I reduce fitness goal to 3x/week—80% confident

8) **I will begin working on the following goal and supporting affirmations:**

I will move (class, walking, gardening) for 30 minutes and meditate for 5 minutes at least 3 days/week for the next month.

9) **Seal the deal with a contract.**

On 9/22 I will begin to self-monitor or journal to evaluate my success in reaching my goal, I will move (class, walking, gardening) for 30 minutes and meditate for 5 minutes at least 3 days/week for the next month, and discuss successes and challenges with members of my workshop class on 10/12.
—Barbara C, 9/21

Additional thoughts or notes:

This feels doable—I don't know how the meditation will help, but I'll try it—what's 5 minutes?

There are a number of additional lifestyle self-assessment tools available that can help you explore more deeply. Several are easily accessible on the Internet at no charge. These are listed in the Resources for Further Study section of this book.

If you have done all the exercises in this chapter, you have quite a dossier on yourself, including the seeds of exploring your lifestyle issues and developing some initial goals. Interpreting all of this "raw data" alone can be daunting, and a nutrition professional or an informed friend may help you prioritize goals and clarify your strategies and barriers.

This clear-eyed self-study (svadhyaya) can also activate emotions such as resistance or self-judgment. If this happens, it is a perfect time to explore yogic exercises for self-discovery. A yoga practice can help you relax and integrate strong emotions and can allow the work you have done to sink in.

Yoga and Meditation Exercises for Self-Discovery

Before launching a new health regimen, talk it over with your physician. If you have an existing medical condition, work with your health team to adapt this work to honor your medical needs. Professional yoga instruction is recommended for beginners.

Wear loose, comfortable clothing that does not inhibit movement for practice. Find a quiet space large enough to stand with wide legs and to move your arms in all directions. A towel or yoga mat and a cushion or blanket can help make you more comfortable.

Principles for safe yoga practice include moving slowly and with awareness, maintaining smooth, easy breathing through the nose unless otherwise instructed, and not straining to achieve a position. Your yoga practice is a time to pay attention to your physical abilities and limitations and to make compassionate adjustments accordingly.

Please note that there are several types of yoga postures not recommended for an overweight body. For example, inversions (going upside-down) facilitate the cleansing processes of the body, which is of particular benefit to those with hypo-digestion (slow digestion in relation to appetite) and the resulting buildup of body mass, toxins, and so forth. But the primary inversions of yoga—headstand and shoulder stand—are invitations for injury for beginners with excess body weight and low muscle strength. So, if you are overweight, especially if you are not regularly physically active, you may need to adjust postures in order for them to be safe and beneficial. But, no matter who you are, each asana (posture) may be done safely with skillful adjustments. For the following practice, I describe modifications for larger bodies. It requires awareness and an attitude of taking your time to cultivate a beneficial practice. If you are not regularly physically active, begin slowly so that you prevent injuries related to overdoing it. One yoga principle says that practicing for 10 minutes every day is preferable to practicing for 3 hours once a week. It's showing up for regular daily practice that holds the magic.

A yoga practice usually contains a period of centering or settling down and turning your awareness inward, warming up or preparing the body for practice, a period of asana (physical postures) with pranayama (awareness to breath and energy movement), and relaxation/integration. There is, however, no "recipe" for a practice, and the elements listed often blend together. A period of meditation often follows a yoga practice.

Exercises 3 through 7 may help you begin a simple home yoga asana (posture) practice. Exercise 8 is a journaling exercise to help you explore the emotional side of self-discovery from a yogic perspective. The insights you glean from your intention and journaling work may help you weave aspects of the yoga practice into your evolving lifestyle plan.

Exercise 3: Centering

Benefits: Centering helps you to slow down and let your whole being arrive on your mat. It begins the process of turning inward and marks your intention of self-study (svadhyaya).

Contraindications: None.

Instructions: Come to a comfortable seated position, either on the floor or in a chair. You can sit on a cushion or folded blanket if that is more comfortable than the floor. If you sit in a chair, keep your back and neck straight and place your feet flat on the floor. Take a little time to arrange yourself comfortably.

Sit up tall with a straight spine. Begin to feel the base of the spine—the bones sometimes called the sitz bones, the tailbone, and the pubic bone—grow heavy and reach down through the chair, blankets, cushions, and floor to the ground beneath the floor. Take a few moments to feel this grounding of the spine. Then begin to notice the thread of your breath. Notice your inhaling and exhaling and see if you can become a bit fascinated, noticing how the nose, throat, chest, and other parts of the body react to the inhale and the exhale. Invite yourself to come into your "yogic space"—a place of non-judging and compassion, a place of non-striving, and a safe place to explore sensation. Perhaps form an intention for your practice—what would you like to bring into your life through this practice?

Exercise 4: A Warm-up: Cat and Dog Breathing

Benefits: A gentle way to move with and become aware of the spine and the breath.

Contraindications: None.

Instructions: Come to your hands and knees in a table position—palms in line under shoulders and knees in line under hips. On the inhale, let the belly inflate toward the floor and let your gaze roll up toward the ceiling, tailbone rolling upward. The spine is scooped in this position, sometimes called the "dog position." On an exhale, round the spine, pressing the belly up toward the ceiling, letting the head hang and the tailbone roll under. This is sometimes called the "cat position," as it is reminiscent of a scared cat arching its back. Move smoothly and slowly between the cat and dog positions with each breath, noticing the movement of the spine, and perhaps noticing if any areas of the spine feel flat or are not participating in the movement. Just notice these areas and see if you can breathe into them. Repeat this series for 5-10 breaths and work up to 3-5 minutes.

Cat and dog breathing looks like this:

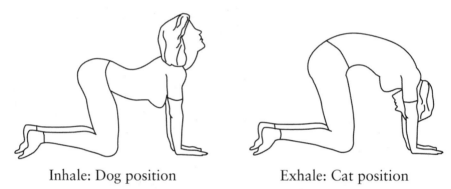

Inhale: Dog position   Exhale: Cat position

Exercise 5: Downward-Facing Dog (Adho Mukha Svanasana)

Benefits: Stretches and strengthens arms, shoulders, legs, and hips; lengthens muscles in back of leg; lengthens the spine. Gentle inversion facilitates the exhale.

Full downward dog may look like this:

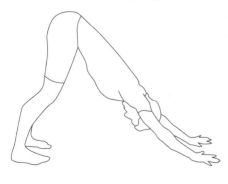

Contraindications: Recent injury of the hands, wrists, or shoulders; glaucoma or uncontrolled high blood pressure. For larger bodies, particularly if arm strength is low, try the modifications described.

Instructions: Begin in the neutral table position, hands directly under the shoulders and knees directly under the hips. Spread your fingers wide with the middle fingers parallel. Press through the index fingers and thumbs, and press the knuckles gently into the floor to keep the weight from grinding into the wrists. Let the upper arm rotate externally so that the shoulders are wide and the chest is open.

Inhale, and on the exhale press into the knuckles and lift the hips high toward the ceiling, keeping the knees bent initially so that you can emphasize the lengthening of the spine. Press the floor away with the hands to give a stretch to the arms. Let the head either release down toward the floor or keep the ears in line with the arms, whichever is more comfortable. Bend one knee while pressing the opposite heel toward the floor to open the back of the legs. Repeat, alternating heels. Draw the belly button in toward the spine. Hold this posture for about 30 seconds if comfortable at first, and work your way up to 2 or 3 minutes. Breathe. Notice where sensations build, and breathe into that area. Inhale, and on the exhale release the knees back to the floor.

Modification 1: If you cannot support the weight of your body on your arms and shoulders, downward-facing dog can be modified to make it more accessible.

Downward-facing dog against the wall may look like this:

Instructions: Face a wall, standing about one leg's distance from the wall. Press down into your feet, and activate your belly by drawing it in toward the spine. Reach your hands

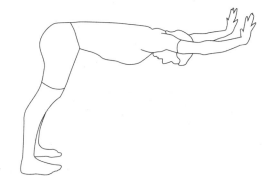

forward and place them, shoulder-width apart, on the wall. Press into your hands and let your shoulders roll down your back. Begin to drop your head between your arms as you lengthen back through your tailbone and continue to draw the belly in. If you want to work deeper, step your feet further back so that more of your weight is in your hands and your active belly holds you. Feel the stretch through your armpit/chest and spine. Take several breaths, and then to release, step forward, activate the belly, and come back to a standing position.

Modification 2: Place a sturdy chair, such as a folding chair, against a wall in such a way that it will not slip. Place palms on the seat of the chair shoulder-width apart. Activate your abdomen by drawing the belly button in toward the spine. Walk slowly backward, allowing your spine to lengthen and your head to come between your upper arms. Hold for 15-30 seconds, slowly working your way up to a minute or two. When you are ready to release, walk forward to the chair and bend your knees, keeping your spine long as you lift your torso to an upright position.

Exercise 6: Full Forward Fold (Uttanasana)

Benefits: Full stretch of the back of the body, to increase awareness there. Passive lengthening of the spine. Muscles in the neck can release. Opens hips. This is a calming posture.

Contraindications: Unregulated high blood pressure or glaucoma. Be especially mindful of keeping your knees bent if you have low back issues.

Forward fold may look like this:

Instructions: Begin in a standing position with your feet hip-distance apart. Look down to make sure that the outsides of the feet are parallel. Lift and spread the toes, then place them back down so that you can see the floor between the toes. (If this doesn't happen naturally with your feet, the more you practice the better you'll get.) Press into the knuckles of the feet at the base of the toes, and press into the center of the heel and feel the arches of the feet lift. Inhale, moving your hands overhead, and take the opposite elbow with each hand. Release your shoulders down away from your ears. Stand up straight, lifting your heart up away from your waist. Activate your abdomen, inhale, and on the exhale extend forward at the hips to a flat back. Bend the knees a bit to make space in the low back. Try to keep the low back lengthening and straight. On the next exhale, fold all the way forward, keeping the knees soft to accommodate the low back. Let the arms (still holding the elbows) hang down. If you feel discomfort in the low back, you can support the back by releasing the elbows and placing your hands on your thighs, coming up a little. If your belly is preventing you from folding, you may want to reach across and move it to one side or in such a way that it is comfortable but does not inhibit your forward movement. If it's comfortable for you, bring your weight into the balls of the feet. Breathe, relax, and stay for 20-30 seconds at first, working up to 2-3 minutes. To release, activate the abdomen and slowly roll up, focusing on the internal sensation.

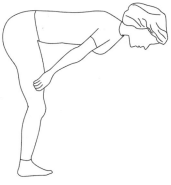

A modified forward fold may look like this:

Modification 1: If you have low back issues, you can keep your hands on your hips rather than reaching them overhead. As you bend forward you can place your hands on your legs for support. You can also place a chair in front of you prior to beginning the exercise to provide more support by holding the chair if your back is not comfortable in a fuller forward fold. Any adjustments in a posture that can help you relax in a posture, and stretch without strain, are helpful. In yoga practice, work near your "yogic edge of comfort." That is, you want to go deep enough into a posture for some stretch and sensation to occur, but not so deep as to cause straining and tensing. Be able to breathe smoothly and comfortably throughout the practice.

Exercise 7: Relaxation (Savasana)

Benefits: Releases tension and calms the body, integrates practice.

Contraindications: None. If lying on your back is not comfortable or possible, other positions in which the body is fully supported and can relax are fine. Other options are lying on your side with pillows under the upper knee and other cushions to support, or sitting in a comfortable chair. Whatever position you can relax into support will work.

Savasana may look like this:

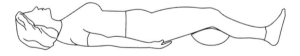

Instructions: Find a comfortable place to lie on the floor. You may roll a blanket and place it under your knees to help release the lower back. If you have an eye pillow (a soft bag often filled with barley hulls or lavender), you can place it over your eyes. Let the palms face up toward the ceiling, and allow the feet to relax. Let the body be fully relaxed, releasing into the floor. Give attention to the breath and scan the body for signs of tension, consciously releasing any holding with each exhale. Let the breath be easy and quiet. Relax (without falling asleep) for 5-10 minutes. To come out of the posture, begin by wiggling your fingers and toes. Bend your knees and slowly roll to one side. Press yourself back up to a comfortable seated position.

Exercise 8: Journaling Questions: Svadhvaya (Self-Study)

Instructions: Take a moment to sit quietly, listening to the flow of your breath. Then, spend time exploring the following questions in your journal.

- What can you feel in your physical body right now?
- What recent experiences (e.g., exercises, struggling with a cold, a hard day at work, or a large meal) can you feel the effects of?
- Describe in detail how an area of your body, or your body as a whole, physically feels right now.

Now relax for a moment. Begin to notice if there is an emotional component to the physical feeling that you just explored. Describe any emotions you feel as you review these physical sensations. Write down whatever comes to mind.

What other emotions are present in your body right now?

Now take a moment to explore your energy level and the quality of your energy right now. Do you feel blue, depressed, or upbeat—content or tired? Again, there is no need to change anything; just explore your energy level and write down anything you notice.

Take another break. Relax. From the work you've done, can you identify the "mental talk" or "mental chatter" (that is, the flow of thoughts, often judgments) separate from the physical sensations or the emotions you've explored? What was your "mental chatter" during these exercises?

A sample program for getting started with tools and exercises described thus far is outlined here. There are many quality yoga books, home-study CD practices, and other resources that can help you get started or support your progress. Check the Resources for Further Study section for ideas.

Sample Program for a Week: Getting Started

- ◆ Do the intention exercises
- ◆ Record your measurement, risk factors, and resources
- ◆ Do the Lifestyle Manifestation exercise
- ◆ Take a beginners' yoga class 1-2x/week
  or
  Do a beginners' yoga CD/DVD practice
  or
  Practice centering, cat and dog breathing, downward-facing dog, forward fold, and relaxation
- ◆ Journal from above experiences, or use the journaling questions 2-3x/week

chapter 4 four

awareness: deepening your reality project

NOW IS THE TIME

*Now is the time to know
That all that you do is sacred...*

*My dear, please tell me,
Why do you still*

*Throw sticks at your heart...
What is it in that sweet voice inside
That incites you to fear?*

*Now is the time for the world to know
That every thought and action is sacred.*

*This is the time
For you to compute the impossibility
That there is anything
But Grace.*

*Now is the season to know
That everything you do
Is sacred.*

—HAFIZ, TRANSLATION BY DANIEL LADINSKY

"My eating disorder started in college—I had a collection of friends who were doing it, and while at first it seemed gross, it was a way of being able to eat without gaining weight," said Christine. "While I kept vowing never to do it again, I kept doing it, and it grew to several times each day. I really don't know why. There are definitely days that I eat normally. It's just not a big deal. I want to eat healthy, and I do. But there are days when I think about food all day, and I eat pure sugar and fat. On those bad-food days, I am definitely more prone to purge after binging. Everything's bad on those days."

Remember the Yoga Sutra, an ancient text made up of deceptively simple phrases, or sutras, that guide the yoga practitioner? The basics of a healthy lifestyle can seem simple too, but we all know they can be difficult to follow in practice.

> **An Eating Sutra**
>
> Eat what you want
>
> When you are hungry
>
> Until you are comfortable.

Eating what you want when you're physically hungry until you are sated is normal healthy eating. It nurtures mental and physical wellness. Healthy eating usually happens at regular times, typically three meals and one or two snacks each day, to satisfy hunger. Healthy eating is regulated by physical internal signals of hunger, appetite, and satiety. According to healthy weight and eating expert Francis Berg, normal healthy eating:

- Enhances your feelings of well-being. You eat for health and energy, pleasure, and to socialize. Afterward, you feel good.
- Provides variety, moderation, and balanced nutrition.

~~⌐ Promotes clear thinking, stable moods, and even performance. It supports healthy relationships in family, work, school, and community. Thoughts of food, hunger, and weight occupy only a small part of the day (perhaps 10-15%).

~~⌐ Nurtures good health, vibrant energy, and healthy growth and development. It promotes a stable weight within a wide range reflecting your genetic background and environment.

In short, it's free of the worry-binge-compensate cycle and compulsiveness that are so easy to fall into in our modern food environment. Our dominant food culture has become very dysfunctional.

How does Berg say normal eating compares with dysfunctional eating?

~~⌐ Dysfunctional or disordered eating patterns are irregular and chaotic (such as with fasting, binging, dieting, or skipping meals), or feature overeating or under-eating much more or less than the body wants or needs. Instead of feeling better after eating, you often feel worse, physically or emotionally, or both.

~~⌐ Feeling fatigued, irritable, moody, chilled, less able to concentrate, and increasingly self-absorbed is common. Thoughts of food, hunger, and weight may occupy 20-65% of waking hours, or more. Potential health problems vary depending on the dysfunction. Risk of developing eating disorders increases.

Internal Awareness:
A Tool for Exploring Emotional Eating

"I'm all about emotional eating," added Barbara. "Food is emotional! I find great comfort in eating, and I know that's going to be a huge cycle to break for me. It's just there, it's so easy, and it works. Finding other things that give me that release…well, maybe food hasn't worked so well, has it? Am I happy overweight and eating like this? Ouch…I guess not."

After exploring these issues for several weeks, Christine said, "My emotional state is definitely a red flag. When I'm feeling tired, or when life feels harder, I need comfort, and food is an easy way to calm myself. So, I'm exploring other things, such as calming baths, napping (an extravagance for me!), or calling supportive friends. That has helped me do less emotional eating and zoning out in front of the TV."

We all get hungry. Hunger for food is a basic human drive. You feel stomach contractions. A dip in energy. And a host of thoughts and signals that nudge you to eat. That's physical hunger.

Unfortunately, emotions often trigger similar sensations. When your appetite and hunger are driven by the stress response, depression, or other psychological issues, the natural hunger-eating interplay often gets uncoupled. Emotional eating is the result.

You can stop the cycle of emotional eating by recognizing your trigger "red flags"—the things in your life that remind you to "wake-up" and pop into witness consciousness.

Witness consciousness

Accessing witness consciousness is the process of bringing the observer within you to bear on your external experience. Cultivating witness consciousness is a means of developing and expanding your body-based intelligence and therefore expanding your consciousness. It is a process that enables you to pause, lift out of the ongoing stream of chatter in your mind (the ego-mind), observe, evaluate, and act from a more non-judgmental global perspective. Psychotherapist and yoga instructor Stephen Cope notes that witness consciousness is similar to the "observing ego" in contemporary Western psychology. From this perspective, nothing is good or bad, it just is.

The ability to access witness consciousness is nothing short of one of the most powerful tools you can learn for behavior change. Psychologists, like yogis, believe that if your witness consciousness is insufficiently developed, you will suffer. Without witness consciousness,

"How about this for an example of unconscious eating?" said Christine. "I love to watch TV with a bowl of popcorn. Sometimes a really big buttery bowl, when I'm tired or have had a bad day. I remember sitting down with my popcorn and, the next thing I know, the bowl is completely empty! I know my lack of awareness of eating is not 'witness consciousness,' but when I wake up and see the empty bowl I realize I've been almost sleep-eating."

your ego-mind—that part of your mind whose role is to make sure you stay safe and make rational choices (but whose reactionary chatter has an opinion on absolutely everything)—rules the roost. When that happens, you tend to become overly identified with thoughts, feelings, and external value systems such as those portrayed in the media and you tend to lose connection with your own real intentions and value system.

Many of us have shared the experience Christine describes—not remembering eating or enjoying food. When you become aware of this eating pattern and begin to explore and possibly alter it, you are using a higher state of consciousness—witness consciousness—to help you examine your behavior.

Witness consciousness is self-observation without judgment. Learning to let go into an open, non-judgmental state is one of yoga's central, and most difficult, lessons. But simply participating in the process—just trying—tends to increase your capacity to access witness consciousness and to release the ego-mind's constant judging. Simply taking the time to be open to it encourages a budding of your deeply aware, attuned intelligence. Here is an exercise to help you explore your witness consciousness:

Exercise 9: Accessing the Witness

Benefits: Stress management, aid to meditation. A tool for developing insight.

Contraindications: If you are unable to lie on the floor, this exercise may be done in a bed or in any position in which you can fully relax.

Instructions: Lie down on the floor in a place where you will not be disturbed for the period of this exercise. Close your eyes, breathe, and relax. Take a few breaths just to soften into the floor. Imagine yourself floating above your body, looking down at yourself. Invite yourself to view this body with ahimsa (compassion, non-violence), or as if this body belonged to a beloved sister, brother, or friend. What would you wish for this beloved being's process of self-care? What feelings do you wish for this person to have about her caring for herself? How might these feelings change her life? From your work with identifying barriers and triggers, what would you say to this beloved being's work on that particular issue?

Bring awareness back into your physical body, stretch gently, and journal on any insights that came from this experience.

Conscious eating

Unconscious overeating is actively promoted in the media, especially in food advertising. Conscious, mindful eating is a simple process that can help deepen your awareness of what and how you eat. It is an eating meditation and builds on your ability to access witness consciousness.

A conscious eating practice can be especially valuable to you if you overeat as an emotional coping mechanism. If you recognized yourself in Christine's experience of eating without being aware of what or how much she is eating or whether she is physically hungry or not, you are a prime candidate for conscious eating practices. Conscious eating promotes awareness and appreciation of the sensory aspects of food: texture, taste, smell, appearance, and sound. And, like most yoga practice, conscious eating gives us the gift of simply slowing down.

As you become a more conscious eater, you develop the skill of recognizing the triggers that lead to your overeating. Triggers may include physical or emotional states (such as sadness, stress, fatigue, or loneliness), environments (e.g., in front of the TV or in the snack room at work), responses to people (such as a relative or friend who encourages overeating as a show of love or support, or

 After practicing conscious eating, Christine said, "I have never eaten as slowly as I ate during the conscious eating meditation. If I could eat everything like that, I'd definitely eat better and a lot less. And, I really tasted my food—it was so good! Slowing down is going to be tough, but I can see the benefits now and I'm going to try to be more conscious."

a friendship built around high-calorie events such as weekly happy hours with fried snacks), or going the whole day without eating and then snacking from dinnertime until bedtime. Becoming a more conscious eater does not mean that your triggers are eliminated; rather, you learn to manage trigger situations with witness consciousness. You can explore and evaluate triggers by the degree to which they undermine normal eating. Then, strategies for addressing a particular trigger may be weighed and tested according to how easy the change would be and how much benefit it would be. This can be challenging work to do on your own; a nutrition professional can play an active role in helping you prioritize triggers, strategizing alternative behaviors, and helping you track progress. As you become more conscious in your eating habits, you'll be able to recognize physical hunger and satiety and to differentiate those physical signals from emotional or habitual signs to eat.

Exercise 10: Conscious Eating Meditation

Benefits: Promotes dietary awareness.

Contraindications: None.

Instructions: Make a conscious decision early in the day to prepare and eat one meal or snack as a meditation. Decide what it will be and when you'll do it. Give yourself a half hour for a snack, and more for a meal.

Prepare your food by hand, preferably without machines, in silence. Simple preparations are great (such as peeling an orange or making a simple salad or sandwich). What can you make that honors and nourishes your body? As you prepare your food, take your time, breathe, and move slowly. Appreciate each ingredient with all five senses. What is its color and texture? How does it smell? Does it have sound? Vibration? Honor the food and yourself with slow and caring preparation.

Once prepared, sit down with your food in front of you. Place both feet on the floor and consciously connect with the ground. Bring the palms of your hands to hover over your food, and notice what you feel. With your palms here, give thanks for the food, the experience, and anything else you are grateful for.

Begin to eat. Again, appreciate the food with all five senses. Chew slowly and completely—can you chew each mouthful 30 or 50 or even 100 times? Explore the full flavor and the variety of tastes that make up this food. Feel the texture, note the smell, and listen to the sound of each bite you take. Place your eating utensils back on the table between each bite of food. Breathe and relax. Once you complete your meal or snack in this way, pause. This may be a good time to note your reflections in your journal.

Breath: The ultimate mind-body tool

Yoga is in large part a practice of breathing. Why all this focus on the breath? Well, it seems that one of your most effective mind-body tools is right under your nose.

Respiration is the only physiological function that is both voluntary and involuntary. Like nutrition, breathing and its impact on health has largely escaped the attention of the mainstream medical community. The effects of how you breathe reach well beyond simply circulating air into and out of your body. Subtle physiological changes in the quality of digestion and molecular energy processes adjust in response to each breath you take. Today scientists are actively investigating what yogis have believed and practiced for centuries—that adjusting your breath may provide a non-invasive means of altering your physiology and psychology.

In the Yoga Sutra, Patanjali explains that the control of life force (prana) is the regulation of the inhalation and the exhalation. Scientists studying yogic respiration suggest that the voluntary control of the depth, duration, and frequency of respiration influence the heart and the vagus nerve, and therefore the autonomic nervous system. The autonomic nervous system contains the sympathetic nervous system, where the "fight or flight" stress response is orchestrated, and the parasympathetic nervous system, which calms us back down after our stress response has been activated.

"Practicing pranayama is easier for me than trying to meditate," said Christine. "I've found I really enjoy feeling the subtleties of my breath expanding through my body, and I like to do the different yogic breathing methods. It feels nourishing."

According to yoga and its medical system, Ayurveda, disease results from an imbalance in the flow of life force (prana). Prana flows through the breath, as well as through other pathways of clearing toxins and ingesting nutrients in their broadest sense, including relationships, environments, and diet.

Watching the influence of emotions on the breath is watching the mind-body dance in full swing. Fear may elicit shallow, rapid breathing; a depressed individual may have a heavy, labored breathing pattern; and a calm person may breathe deeply and slowly.

Yogis suggest that the breath-based relationship between the body and mind is a two-way street; that is, if a certain state of mind results in a particular breathing pattern, then adopting a particular breathing pattern may illicit a certain state of mind. The study of relationships between emotion and breathing patterns is a hot area of clinical and behavioral research. So far, scientists are finding that there seems to be a relationship between breath and emotion, and it can be a two-way street, but the relationship is complex. You might breathe fast and heavily, for example, in response to both positive and negative emotions. Capturing and quantifying that silken life-thread of the breath is proving elusive.

Yoga uses attention to the breath as a means of providing the mind something to focus on—a job to do. That helps you draw your attention inward. Here are several basic yoga breathing techniques that may help you add pranayama (breath and energy awareness) to your yoga and meditation practice. Dirgha pranayama and ujjayi pranayama may be done either seated or in yoga asana (postures).

Exercise 11: Yogic Breathing Techniques

Benefits: Stress management, aids meditation.

Contraindications: For those with bronchitis and other pulmonary issues, and for women who are pregnant, perform all breathing exercises very gently. Strong or forceful breathing exercises are not recommended for these individuals.

Instructions:

Centering and finding the breath

Find a comfortable seated position where you can sit up straight, either in a chair with your feet flat on the floor or on the floor seated on a cushion or blanket with your pelvis tipped slightly forward so that your spine can lengthen upward. Take a moment to notice how you are feeling mentally and physically. Listen to and feel your breath. Locate and visualize breathing into the area of your heart.

Dirgha pranayama: A calming yogic breath

On an inhale, allow your belly to expand. On the exhale, let your belly release, pressing it gently in toward your spine. Exhale completely. Breathe slowly. On the next inhale, breathe into the belly, then into the mid-belly, and finally into the chest. Release the breath from the top down; so first release the chest, then the mid-belly, and finally the lower belly, with a little drawing in toward the spine at the end of the exhale. Don't force or push the breath; just let it flow as if in response to an invitation. You might imagine that your body is a vessel that you are filling and emptying with breath.

Ujjayi pranayama: Extends, deepens, and evens breath

Press the glottis (palate) softly against the back of the throat, which will narrow the air passage there. This action in the throat is the same as if you were fogging a mirror. Inhale and exhale in this position, making a soft "haaa" sound in the back of your throat. This breath is also called "the ocean sounding breath" because of the gentle wavelike sound it makes.

Lifestyle journaling

Keeping a lifestyle journal is a tried-and-true method of exploring habits. It can be challenging, but as with anything, you get out of it what you put in. For this program, your lifestyle journal can reflect the emotive aspect of eating, your exploration of physical activity, and awareness coming from yoga and meditation. Exercise 12 gives an example that may guide you in setting up your own lifestyle journal. Remember, too, that your lifestyle journal for a particular day or week will reflect what you are working on for that period of time.

Exercise 12: Lifestyle Journal

Name: _____ Date: _____

Nutrition goal for the day: _____

_____

Record everything you eat and drink, being as specific as possible (ex., ¼ cup oatmeal with ¼ cup 1% milk and 2 tsp. honey). Also note your physical activity, meditation/yoga practice, and any "eating triggers" you notice. Be as specific and complete as possible.

Time	Food eaten	Amount	Physically hungry? 1, 2, 3*	Mood before eating	Where & with whom	Ate in response to...

*1 = not hungry, 2 = hungry, 3 = very hungry

Goal met? _____ If not, what were the barriers to meeting your goal?

_____

_____

_____

Did you notice any "eating triggers" other than physical hunger? _____

_____

Meditation/yoga practice consisted of: _____

_____

Physical activity today—activity and time spent: _____

_____

_____

_____

Did you notice any barriers to your meditation, yoga, or physical activity? _____

Any ideas on how you might address the barriers you identified? _____

_____

_____

Comments/insights: _____

_____

_____

_____

_____

Use your journal and your yoga/meditation practice to explore barriers and eating triggers. Remember that we all have barriers to a healthy lifestyle, and it is a matter of finding what works for you.

Here is a sample of Christine's Lifestyle Journal:

Name: _____ *Christine* _____ Date: *September 25*

Nutrition goal for the day: _____ *Not to eat after dinner* _____

_____

Record everything you eat and drink, being as specific as possible (ex., ¼ cup oatmeal with ¼ cup 1% milk and 2 tsp. honey). Also note your physical activity, meditation/yoga practice, and any "eating triggers" you notice. Be as specific and complete as possible.

Time	Food eaten	Amount	Physically hungry? 1, 2, 3*	Mood before eating	Where & with whom	Ate in response to...
7 AM	Coffee, w/ milk, sugar	1c, 1tsp ea	1	Tired	Kitchen, alone	Habit
noon	Turkey sand on wheat, let, tom, mayo	2oz. meat, 2 sl bread, 2 sl tom, 1tbs	2	Hungry	Work, alone	Hungry
2 PM	2 Candy bar, bag of chips	12 oz, large bag	Starving, 3	Tired and hungry, aggravated	Car, alone	Starving
6 PM	Spaghetti with sauce, meatballs	Lots—2 plates full, 4 big meatballs	2	Tired, sad	Kitchen, alone	Dinner time
8 PM	Popcorn with butter	5-10 cups	1	Bored, tired	Bed, alone	TV, bored

*1 = not hungry, 2 = hungry, 3 = very hungry

Goal met? __N__ If not, what were the barriers to meeting your goal?
I was tired and frustrated today—and skipped my physical activity

_____

_____

Did you notice any "eating triggers" other than physical hunger? _____
Definitely—when I'm tired I'm easily sidetracked. Overeating in the car, and in the evening were problems too.

Meditation/yoga practice consisted of: _____
5 min meditation in the morning

Physical activity today—activity and time spent: _____
Skipped it!

Did you notice any barriers to your meditation, yoga, or physical activity? _____ *Yes!* _____

Any ideas on how you might address the barriers you identified? _____
_____ *Better planning* _____

Comments/insights: _*I need to find ways to overcome resistance*_ _____
*when I have challenging days* _____

_____

_____

Body awareness meditations

There are many different methods that can support your meditation practice. Each method uses a slightly different focus, but they are all, in the end, tricks to help the mind settle down. Psychologist Lawrence LeShan, scholar and teacher Richard Miller, and others have developed some beautiful body-based meditations. Here are two body awareness meditations that you may use for your daily meditation or on occasion.

Exercise 13: Encircling Light—Body Scan Meditation

Benefits: Stress management, body awareness. Aids meditation.

Contraindications: None.

Instructions: Find a quiet, comfortable place to sit in meditation. You can sit in a chair or on the floor. If you are in a chair, uncross your legs and place both feet on the floor. Take a few centering breaths, and allow your awareness to focus on your breath. Resist changing the breath; just observe it.

Imagine a benevolent beam or bead of light sitting at the center of your navel. Very slowly, allow the beam to circumnavigate your waist. Then, allow the beam to circle to your right waist. Let the beam travel down the outer right hip and down the outside of your right leg. Then, allow the beam to travel slowly across the sole of your right foot, up the inside of the right leg, and down the inseam of the left leg. Let the beam travel across the left sole and up the outer left leg. Then, allow the beam to head up to the left armpit, down the inner left arm, and onto the left palm. Let the beam slowly track across the webbing between the thumb and first finger to the top of the hand, and continue up the outer arm to the shoulder. Let the beam slowly travel across the shoulder, head up the left side of the neck and around the head, and down the right side of the neck. Let the beam continue in this manner around the right arm, to the right armpit, down the right waist, and return to the navel. Let the light begin to expand from the center of your navel, and the center of your being. Let your entire body be bathed by the light emanating from your own center.

"During the encircling light meditation, I couldn't feel my waist at all," said Christine. "But my heart was really calling to be encircled, so my beam went there...twice. In reflecting on it, I am really unconscious of my belly, and I definitely have a hungry heart! So my goals in my Lifestyle Manifestation are all around learning how to feed my body with food, and my heart and emotions with other things."

Deepen your breath, and slowly open your eyes. Take note of any areas in your body that you could not feel. This is not at all unusual; just take note. As you practice this and other body-centered meditation, your awareness in those areas will increase.

Exercise 14: Healing Waters—Body Awareness Meditation

Benefits: Stress management, body awareness, aid to meditation.

Contraindications: None.

Instructions: Find a quiet, comfortable place to sit in meditation. It can be in a chair or on the floor. If you are in a chair, uncross your legs and place both feet on the floor. Take a few centering breaths, and allow your awareness to focus on your breath. Resist changing the breath; just observe it.

Bring your awareness to one area of your body—one where you think healing may be needed. Focus on that area and begin to imagine it filling with healing water. Note the temperature, texture, smell, and beautiful color and light of the water. Notice how that area of your body feels when it is filled and massaged with healing fluid. Envision toxins in that area of the body, including physical substances as well as emotions of fear, sadness, and pain, flowing into the water. Then allow the water to slowly drain away, taking the toxins with it, leaving you clear and refreshed. Repeat this three times. Note how the area, and how your whole body, feels.

Exercise 15: Journaling: Ahimsa (Non-violence)

Benefits: Stress management, aids behavior change.

Contraindications: None.

Instructions: Prepare to journal by finding a comfortable, quiet place. Take a moment to quiet and center yourself.

1) Are there times when your eating represents violence to your own body, either by under- or overeating, or something else? Describe an example in your journal.

In the above example, can you recall what you were feeling before, during, and after the episode? What was your physical body seeking in the experience? What was your emotional body seeking? Mental body?

2) Can you think of another activity or way of being in response to your body's needs that may be more compassionate?

3) What happens, emotionally, as you invite yourself to be more compassionate toward yourself? How does that feel in your physical body?

"There is no way that I can do these exercises and not change what and how and why I eat!" said Christine. "I can see that I have a lot of work to do in my head, but also, my habits are shifting just from paying attention."

4) Do you have a body weight goal? When was the last time you weighed that number? Do you believe this number is realistic for *your* body and *your* life right now?

5) Are you willing and able to make the life adjustments to attain that weight? How does holding this ideal number in your mind feel? Does it impact your self-esteem and respect? Is there another goal or image that is more compassionate and life-affirming?

6) Describe your best physical feature in detail—what is beautiful about it? As you journal about your own beauty, notice how you feel—physically, emotionally, and energetically.

Sample Plan: Building on Lessons Learned

- Review the Lifestyle Manifestation worksheet, and update as needed

- Witness Consciousness exercise

- Take a beginners' yoga class 1-2x/week
  or
  Do a beginners' yoga CD/DVD practice
  or
  Practice centering, cat and dog breathing, downward-facing dog, forward fold, and relaxation

- Conscious Eating exercise 1-2x/week

- Body Awareness meditation 2-3x/week

- Journal from above experiences, or use journaling questions 2-3x/week

chapter **5** five

change: the art and science of transformation

This Soul of mine within the heart is smaller than a grain of rice, or a mustard seed...; this Soul of mine within the heart is greater than the earth, greater than the sky, greater than the universe. Containing all works, containing all desires, containing all odors, containing all tastes...Whatever is in the macrocosm is in the microcosm also.

— CHANDOGYA UPANISHAD

Both medical science and Eastern philosophy tell us that change is the only constant. But our physical body and human psyche strive for constancy and stability. Becoming aware of the ongoing adjustments your body makes to maintain homeostasis can be a lesson in flowing through life and may give you insight into the way you live.

A central tenet of Eastern philosophies is acceptance of the temporary nature of physical existence. In the grand scheme, one lifetime is a blink of an eye. But letting go of our clinging to life in whatever form that may take, and releasing the habituated need for things to

"With being overweight all my life, and the bias I've felt because of that, I've developed a tough exterior," said Anita. "And while on some levels that has helped me to do the things I have, it has also made me sort of rigid about changing. I'm the strong defiant one, but I realize that one of the things I've been defending is my right not to eat well or take care of myself physically. I can change that."

remain as we imagine they should be, is a major psychological shift for most Westerners.

How We Change

We all know of a habit or two that we could change to become healthier, but we just can't seem to make the shift. Why can't we do it? Because change isn't easy. It isn't comfortable. But as Spencer Johnson describes so well in his book *Who Moved My Cheese?*, change is always going to happen. We all need to learn how to recognize and deal with change in order to be reasonably well adjusted to our modern lives. And the nature of change, unfortunately, is to accelerate. So if you think things are changing faster and faster, you're right.

"I know I don't like change," said Anita. "I love routine and am most productive when my life has a rhythm to it. And I know that I play it safe—in part because I know that will mean less change. I know that if I take more risk and get better at rolling along with change, I'll be happier and probably more successful in some ways. Maybe my love of the status quo is clinging to life. I never really thought of it that way."

With so much change going on, you know that there are scientists studying it. And there are scientists studying how humans change our habits. The resulting behavioral theories are paradigms of change—views into how change usually happens and what can support or undermine the ability to change. Lifestyle counselors often use behavior theories to help people re-frame an issue, or to help them develop new approaches to old issues.

Let's look at just one of the behavior change models. The Stages of Change Model, developed by Prochanska and others, is often used by counselors to guide an individual interested in changing. Chart 10 outlines the model and the strategies a lifestyle counselor may use based on your stage of change with regard to the habit in question.

Chart 10: Stages of Change Model

Stage of Change	Is when you are ...	A counselor may help you move along the continuum by ...
Pre-contemplation	Unaware of the problem and have not thought about change	Increasing your awareness of the need to change, personalizing information on risks and benefits
Contemplation	Thinking about change	Motivating and encouraging you to make specific plans
Planning	Making a plan to change	Assisting in developing concrete action plans, setting gradual goals
Action	Implementing specific action plans	Assisting with feedback, problem solving, social support, reinforcement
Maintenance	Continuing the new habit, or repeating periodic recommended steps	Assisting in coping, reminders, finding alternatives, avoiding slips/relapses

This is just one model. It's one way to think about the process of change.

> "Changing the way I think of taking care of myself has really helped me to get started," said Anita. "In my planning, for the goal I set out of exercising, I can see that doing the manifestation exercises moved me from contemplation, where I just thought to myself once in a while…oh, I should exercise more, to…here's what I can do. And now the reason for doing it is internal—as a means of protecting and loving myself."

In the Stages of Change Model, it is important to realize that maintenance is dynamic and naturally includes relapses, but that each relapse informs a new contemplation-action-maintenance cycle. We never really reach that one perfect moment when we have unequivocally achieved maintenance. So, the process of change is a spiral, as in Chart 11, rather than a straight line, and by learning from lapses the spiral of change progresses.

Chart 11: The Spiral of Change

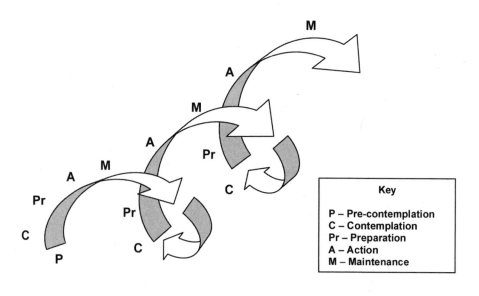

Key

P – Pre-contemplation
C – Contemplation
Pr – Preparation
A – Action
M – Maintenance

Your Behavior Change Strategies

Building on the insights you have gained thus far, the following strategies may help you move along your spiral of change. Some strategies will work better for you than others. Can you use your intuition to guide you on which strategy to try first? Different strategies work in different situations, so as your overall awareness deepens through your yoga and meditation practice, your ability to recognize your triggers and the strategies that work will increase.

"When taking care of myself is more about getting back up when I mess up than being perfect from the start, it's a big pressure relief," said Christine. "And it makes these huge shifts I'm making—learning to work with strong emotions, breaking the binge-purge cycle—feel possible."

Now, we'll explore a number of strategies you may try. Start with the ones that appeal to you the most. The more you practice, the better at positive change you'll get.

Identify non-food rewards

Identifying motivators, rewards, and sources of comfort to replace emotional eating can help you in the contemplation, action, or maintenance phase.

Your non-food rewards may be as simple as taking time to call a friend, taking a bath, or buying a fun new color nail polish. Or it might be changing a hairstyle, scheduling a massage or bodywork session, taking a yoga weekend workshop, or working toward a fitness goal such as a hiking trip. Think about what makes you feel good, what you find comforting, and what you'd like to bring more of into your life. When developing this list it may be helpful to include rewards that do not cost money, so that the reward system does not become entangled with an attachment to material things, which creates problems of its own. Remember, too, that for many of us, taking

"I've definitely used food as comfort," said Anita. "But there are non-food things that comfort me. I love flowers, good novels, or just to take some time to get outside on a nice day. And you know, I wish I could connect with my old friends more. I could definitely give these things to myself as rewards."

"You know, I haven't thought about this in a long time," added Tom, "but I've always loved to surf and I just can't get out there because of problems with my neck. I know other guys who get out there in different ways, but I've always been sort of a purist. I think my reward for giving up the doughnut life will be to explore how a geezer like me can get back out into the surf and have fun."

time to help others is a wonderful reward. Giving away your love doesn't deplete your stock, but actually makes it grow.

The liberal use of rewards, both for achieving your goals and for the times you don't reach a goal but remain in the cycle of change, is a practice with the potential to help you break negative mindsets, particularly if you have the tendency toward the binge-deprivation cycle. If you're someone who isn't sure what it means to be good to yourself, this is a practice for you. The practice of rewarding yourself consciously and lovingly soon becomes simply taking good care of yourself. It feels great and makes you healthier.

Here is an exercise to help you develop your list of non-food rewards.

Exercise 16: Change Boosters: Non-food Rewards

Benefits: Creates awareness of simple ways to self-motivate and finds alternatives to food rewards.

Contraindications: None.

Instructions: Find a quiet place to journal. Take a moment to settle in and to calm your breath. Close your eyes, and begin to think about the things you love to do, the places you love to go, and the people you love to be with. Begin to make a list of each, including how these things or people might be a reward you could give to yourself. Take a look at your list. Are there several things on your list that are free? If not, can you think of a couple of things to add that are free? A few examples may be walks in the woods, taking a bath, connecting with a friend, or doing volunteer work. One way to use these rewards is to incorporate them into goals. For example:

Goal: For the next week, I will eat five servings of fruits or vegetables every day. When I do this, I will reward myself by seeing a new movie with a friend.

Contingency Planning

Contingency planning is learning to be resilient. It's preparing for a rainy lifestyle day. When your yoga class is sold out, when you're starving and there's nothing healthy to eat for miles, when you are traveling on business and there's a bounty of high-calorie social events—a little planning can prevent these challenges from being lifestyle disasters. So, as barriers to reaching your goals come forward and are explored, you find ways to be healthy despite your challenge, or to not lose too much ground. You did contingency planning in the Steps to Successful Lifestyle Manifestation exercise when you thought about ways to address your challenges. Over

"Non-food rewards are a great contingency plan for me," said Anita after several weeks. "It's been a big shift in the way I treat myself, and it's made my life a lot more fun. I still struggle, but now I have some things to help me through."

time, you will develop a safety net of ideas for addressing your most frequent and most challenging situations. Over time, the process of contingency planning will become automatic.

Exploring Negative Thoughts

We all have attitudes and beliefs that underlie the things we do. The negative stress cycle, originally developed by Dr. Herb Benson and his team at Harvard, is described in Chart 12 and shows you how self-limiting beliefs can literally make you sick.

Chart 12: The Negative Stress Cycle

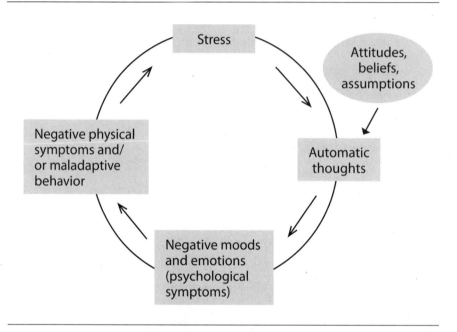

The negative stress cycle is fed by self-limiting automatic thoughts, which are part of the ongoing dialogue running through your mind. These thoughts are deeply rooted in your psyche and are the result of conditioning messages you received from your family and others involved in your early life. In yoga philosophy, these impressions are called samskara, and they are like little pebbles (and a few big boulders!) in the river of your energy channels. The way to clear the pebbles is through the practice of yoga and meditation.

Everyone has samskara—self-limiting or irrational ideas, assumptions, beliefs, and distortions. However, not everyone recognizes them as the mental frames they often are. When you are able to identify self-limiting beliefs, you can then explore the underlying reasons for

"Yes, I definitely have a lot of deep negative mental baggage about eating and about my own self-worth," said Anita. "And it's going to take more than a yoga class once a week to untangle—it's a long-term project. Who knows if I'll ever really get over that early family stuff. But I'm feeling that I can work to uncouple these deep negative feelings from the way I eat and take care of myself. And just practicing taking better care of myself has made me feel better about myself and see that it is possible to change."

them and begin the process of replacing self-limiting patterns with affirmations, intentions, and thoughts that support positive behaviors and break the negative stress cycle.

Yoga, a science of self-awareness, is a tool to help you identify self-limiting thoughts, and through the use of the yamas and niyamas, identify a mindset more supportive of positive lifestyle habits. Remember that your samskara are neither good nor bad. They just are. Chart 13 provides a list of common self-limiting thoughts that Benson and others suggest may play into the negative stress cycle. Do any of them sound familiar?

Chart 13: Common Self-Limiting Thoughts

Limiting Ideas, Assumptions, and Beliefs

- It is an absolute necessity for all adults to have love and approval from peers, family, and friends.
- You must be unfailingly competent and almost perfect in all you undertake.
- It is horrible when people and things are not the way you would like them to be.
- Certain people are evil, wicked, and villainous, and should be punished.
- External events cause more human misery—people simply react as events trigger their emotions.

- You should feel fear and anxiety about anything that is unknown, uncertain, or potentially dangerous.
- It is easier to avoid than to face life's difficulties and responsibilities.
- You need something other or stronger or greater than yourself to rely on.
- The past has a lot to do with determining the present.
- Happiness can be achieved by inaction, passivity, and endless leisure.

Distortions

- "All or nothing" thinking. (Ex.: A client who says she failed because she ate one serving of an unhealthy food, so stopped following her healthy eating plan)
- Overgeneralization. Seeing a negative event as a pattern of defeat. (Ex.: A client who believes she cannot be happy *and* follow a healthy lifestyle)
- Mental filtering. Dwelling only on the negative. (Ex.: A client who followed an overall healthy diet but only focused on the ice cream she had with family)
- Discounting the positive. (Ex.: "You're only saying that to be nice.")
- Jumping to conclusions. Assuming. Mind reading or fortune telling (anticipatory anxiety). (Ex.: "I know I can't do that.")
- Magnification. Exaggerating negative events or minimizing positive traits. (Ex.: "I just can't take it anymore," "My talent is no big deal," "I'm fat.")
- Emotional reasoning. (Ex.: "I feel inadequate, therefore I am inadequate.")
- "Should" statements. These breed pressure and resentment. (Ex.: "I should eat better and exercise more.")

～ Labeling. Name-calling. (Ex.: "He's a loser, a pig. I'm fat, a cow.")

～ Personalization and blame. Assuming responsibility when you weren't responsible. Blaming others for your own negative thoughts or feelings. (Ex.: "He makes me feel this way, and then I eat.")

Exercise 17 will guide you in exploring your interior landscape.

Exercise 17: Negative Stress Cycle Exploration

Benefits: Aids behavior change by identifying self-limiting beliefs.

Contraindications: None, but this exercise is best done in a spirit of compassion, rather than self-judgment.

Instructions: Find a quiet place to write in your journal, and then take a moment to relax and pay attention to your breath. We all have self-limiting assumptions, beliefs, and attitudes. Which of the self-limiting beliefs and distortions listed in the negative stress cycle in Chart 13 seem to describe your thinking? Can you begin to re-frame those beliefs in a way that seems believable? Which beliefs seem most ingrained...which feel as though they'll never change?

During the day, see if you can notice self-limiting beliefs and attitudes as they arise. When your mind makes a negative comment, see if you can re-frame the negative thought into a positive one. Remember,

"Oh yes," said Anita. "I'm a total all-or-nothing thinker. And I've had pretty solid ideas as to how things are: I'll always be overweight and therefore unhealthy, and deep down I think that I've accepted that I'll die fairly young because of my obesity. But through this process, I'm reexamining all of this stuff, trying to sort out what's real and what's my own projection. I'm not doing it alone; I've started some work with a great psychologist Annie recommended. Talk about transformation...I am becoming a completely different person, or uncovering who I really am, and that's a good thing."

we all have negative thoughts. It's part of being human. But, if we can begin to see when and how our negative thoughts impact our behavior negatively, it can shed light on the underlying structure holding poor health habits in place.

Exploring Resistance

As you proceed along the behavior change continuum, you will undoubtedly encounter resistance. Resistance is the dark side of change and is a natural part of the process. Self-doubt or other negative thoughts are bound to pop up. Perhaps those around you will be resistant to losing their snack buddy, or will not want to participate in healthy behaviors and be angry at you for changing. They may experience your change as a judgment against them.

"As you might imagine, my family has had some resistance," said Anita. "But I have these friends who are angels around me to support this transformation, and I'm hoping that when my family sees the change in me, that will give them permission to change too."

Resistance can be powerful and can either derail you or become a key learning experience. In the weight management literature there is much discussion of the psychological benefits of being overweight, including the ability to "hide out" and use overeating for dealing with difficult emotions and for self-comfort. Most of the benefits of overweight and poor health habits, however, are short term and carry big long-term consequences. Your perceptions of your appearance have far-reaching effects upon your identity, so when your body size and appearance begins to change, there is often a period of questioning, resistance, and even crisis.

Resistance takes many forms, and each of us has our own unique ways of resisting change. Active resistance is in when something physically stands in your way, or when you consciously "give up" and make a beeline for the refrigerator. Then there is passive resistance, as in the quiet rationalizations the mind makes for not practicing healthy behaviors.

Yoga practice provides an outlet for exploring this transition to more conscious thinking. As a senior Kripalu yoga teacher says, "Yoga activates and yoga integrates." The yogic practices of dharana (focused concentration), and the niyama of tapas (austerity, passion, heat), may empower you to overcome the obstacle of passive resistance. Exercises in this chapter will help you work with these yogic principles.

Another method for working with resistance and strong emotions is to "ride the wave," described in Chapter Six.

Floating on breath: Salutation to the sun

Salutation to the sun (surya namaskar) is part of many yoga classes, and some styles of yoga are built around this base. I have been in many yoga classes where this flow was taught without awareness...then it can be a monotonous and injury-provoking experience. However, it is also often taught skillfully, with attention to alignment and adaptations for each individual's strengths and limitations. When taken in this light, surya namaskar can be a beautifully simple tool for experiencing the interplay of breath and movement, the dance of will and surrender, and the building of yogic heat (a physical form of tapas).

Here I've described how you can do it and made suggestions for modifications. Another means of building yogic heat through pranayama (energy awareness and control) is a stomach-pumping breathing exercise also included here. Stomach pumping is not only wonderful for building heat, but it also increases belly awareness. Stomach pumping is a great little cleansing activity that makes a nice morning shower ritual.

Exercise 18: Salutation to the Sun (Surya Namaskar)

Benefits: Overall body toner. Excellent for exploring breath with movement. Provides moderate to vigorous physical activity, which you may easily modify for your own level of physical exertion and to accommodate strengths and limitations.

Contraindications: If you have a recent shoulder injury, avoid sections of this exercise where the weight is directly on the arms, as in push-up, plank, or downward dog position. If you have low back pain, keep the knees bent when folding forward. For large bodies with weak arms, this flow can be done in a chair or facing a wall; use a wall for support when folding forward. Downward dog can be performed with the accommodation described in Chapter Three.

Here's how the flow of surya namaskar may look:

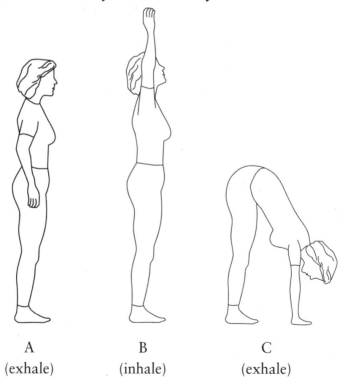

A	B	C
(exhale)	(inhale)	(exhale)

Instructions:

1) Stand with the roots of your big toes together, heals an inch or so apart. Lift your toes and spread them wide, then place them back on the floor. Root the feet into the floor while lifting the arches. Stand tall, draw the belly button gently in toward the spine, and reach the crown of the head up toward the ceiling. Relax your shoulders down your back and feel your collar bones drift away from one another (posture A). Breathe. Exhale, and on an inhale lift your arms up over your head, keeping the shoulders releasing down (posture B).

2) On the exhale, bend the knees slightly and swan-dive forward, keeping the belly engaged and the spine long. Come all the way down to full forward fold (uttanasana, posture C).

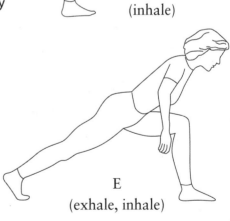

D
(inhale)

3) Inhale, come to a flat back, resting your hands on your thighs, belly engaged, and extending through the crown of your head (posture D).

4) On an exhale, step back with the right leg to a lunge position (posture E), so that the right leg is straight, heel up, and the left knee is bent and over the left heel. Look to see that the left knee is

E
(exhale, inhale)

lined up with the middle of the left foot, both facing straight forward. Let the left knee float right over the left heel. Keep the shoulders gently moving down your back. Be active in the back leg, square the hips (left hip moves gently back), and lengthen the back body from the tailbone through the crown on the head. Inhale, preparing to move.

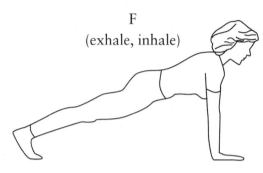

F
(exhale, inhale)

5) Roll your shoulders down your back, place your hands on the floor, and on an exhale step the left foot back to meet the right in a plank position (posture F). Lengthen the body from the crown of the head right down to the heels. Be active in the legs, imagining your inner groins lifting toward the ceiling. Let the abdomen be strong and engaged. Inhale, and on the exhale release your knees, then your chest, then chin to the floor with control, keeping the abdomen strong, the shoulders releasing down the back, chest wide, and elbows in close to the body

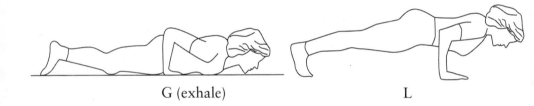

G (exhale)   L

(position G). As you get stronger, you may lower your body from the plank position down to a push-up position (chaturanga dandasana, position L). When you do lower down, keep the shoulders integrated into the back (moving away from the ears) and your chest wide.

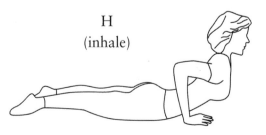

H
(inhale)

6) Place the tops of your feet on the floor, feet hip-width apart and little toes pressing into the mat. Reach down through the toes, activate the legs, and press the pelvis into the floor. Place your palms into the floor at the midline of the chest right along the side of the body with your elbows in line with your palms. Exhale, and on the inhale press the pelvis down as you lift the chest forward and up, rolling the shoulders back, coming into the cobra pose (bhujangasana, posture H). Lengthen the front and the back of the neck evenly.

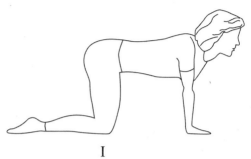

7) Inhale, and on the exhale roll the toes under, press your hips up to a table position (posture I), and then lift your hips up and back to downward-facing dog (adho mukha svanasana, posture J), making sure to keep the shoulders integrated into the back by keeping them wide and moving toward your hips.

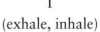

I
(exhale, inhale)

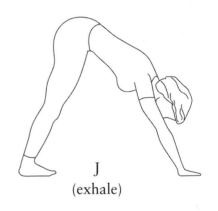

J
(exhale)

8) Take five or six breaths in downward-facing dog, working the posture, noticing where there is constriction, and working to consciously relax those areas.

9) Exhale, and on the inhale step the right foot forward into a lunge (posture K). Square the hips, drawing

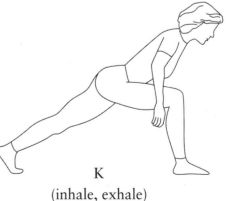

K
(inhale, exhale)

the right hip gently back. Lengthen through the back heel and the crown of the head.

10) Exhale, and on the inhale step the back foot forward. Come up to a flat back, lengthening your body from the tailbone through the crown of the head on the inhale. Exhale into full forward fold (uttanasana, posture C).

11) Pressing into the feet, keeping a slight bend in the knees and the abdomen active, inhale, bringing the arms out to the side and then overhead to draw yourself up to standing.

12) Slowly exhale, bringing the arms down to your side.

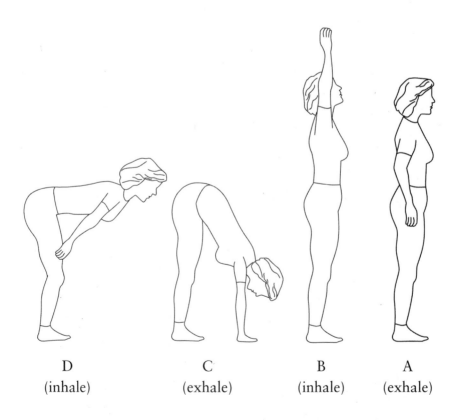

D	C	B	A
(inhale)	(exhale)	(inhale)	(exhale)

Modifications for surya namaskar (salutation to the sun):

Here is what using a wall to modify a portion of surya namaskar may look like:

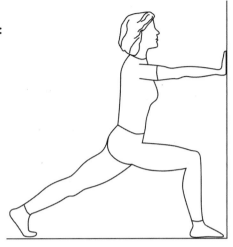

If surya namaskar is too strenuous, or if you are not flexible or strong enough to step back into a lunge from a forward fold, you can do this exercise facing a wall. As you dive forward, place your hands on the wall or on a chair against the wall as in the modification for downward-facing dog presented in Chapter Three. Step one leg back into a gentle lunge, using either the chair or the wall to support you. Then carefully step back to the modified downward-facing dog. If you are using this modification, skip the plank pose and bhujangasana in this flow and move from downward dog to a lunge on the second side; then, inhale with a step forward, and exhale into uttanasana with knees slightly bent. Continue to use the wall for support and to gently strengthen the shoulders, abdomen, and legs. Proceed gently, and experiment with the combination of floor and chair support that enables you to be comfortable and stable while having flowing movement.

Take rest in savasana.

"I love that I can take my yoga practice wherever I go," said Anita. "If I'm traveling, I can do it in my hotel room. And the modifications make the practice work for me. Learning to breathe, learning salutation to the sun… these are great tools that I'll use from here on out."

Finding your fire: The mind-belly connection

The Western beauty ideal has a flat belly and washboard abs. Clothes are designed to girdle the gut, or to hide it. We often try to make the belly simply go away, and many of us feel badly if our bellies do anything but. Controlling our bellies is our outward sign of self-control, and if we cannot, we often feel shame or guilt.

In yoga and other Eastern systems, however, your belly is the very center of your energetic system. It is a key access point to your spiritual wisdom. Western yoga borrows the Japanese term *hara* to describe the belly and its transpersonal power. Does the Buddha have washboard abs? Most definitely not.

Recent discoveries in human biology add fuel to the fire of just how important your belly is. Did you know that the second highest level of neurotransmitters, the chemicals found in the brain and nervous system that carry thoughts and emotion, are found in the gut? This "gut brain," known as the enteric nervous system, appears to reach deep into our evolutionary past. It came way before the one in our head in evolutionary terms, and it's definitely not a center for higher reasoning. The belly's brain responds on the intuitive, nonverbal, instinctual level. When you "feel it in your gut," you're feeling with your gut brain. When you are upset about something, do you have gastrointestinal symptoms such as gas or diarrhea? If you do, you are experiencing how your gut brain can impact digestion. Holding tension in the belly is common, and learning to release that tension and relax the belly is, for those who struggle with weight and eating, an impressive yogic feat.

Western scientists ponder the French Paradox, wherein people in France seem to follow a diet rich in high-fat unhealthy foods yet have low incidence of heart disease and other chronic illness. We've worked so hard to quantify their diet to determine the chemicals that explain the difference. How Western of us! Not until very recently have we looked at *how* they eat rather than (or in addition to) *what* they eat.

And the French eat very differently than we do. Their meals can take hours of relaxed conversation with friends. They enjoy their food with all five senses, allowing their gut brain to prepare their bodies to digest and making mealtime a sensory feast. Think of that way of eating as opposed to our Western "tear the package open and eat it in the car on the way to a meeting" mealtime mentality and you might see why our bodies don't respond as well. How you eat may be just as important, nutritionally, as what you eat.

Many Westerners have done their best to disconnect from the very center of their energy system: their belly. The way we stand, with the belly either drooping forward or sucked back, doesn't take advantage of its ability to stabilize our frames. Yoga provides many ways of developing the aware-

"Annie has worked with me a lot to help me take my eating out of the closet," Anita told the others in the workshop. *"Slowing down, enjoying my food, and finding ways to make meals relaxed and social have been big shifts. I ate everywhere but at the table!"*

ness of our belly, of relaxing so that when we engage it we do so without tension. Learning to harness the power of your belly can profoundly and permanently improve the way you move. If you have ever taken a Pilates class, you have experienced an entire system (derived in part from yogic principles) around activating and using the central core of the body. Pilates is very effective because it dives right in to the impact zone—the hara, the belly.

Exercise 19: Stomach-Pumping Breath

Benefits: Creates internal heat, "wakes up" the stomach. May aid digestion and tone the abdominal muscles.

Contraindications: Recent abdominal surgery, dizziness, or shortness of breath.

Instructions: Begin by lying down or finding a position to relax in for a few moments. With each exhale, see if you can relax the belly a little more. See if you can notice tension in your belly, and consciously release it. Then roll to one side, sit up slowly, and make your way to standing.

Stage 1: Stand with your feet hip-width apart. Root through the feet by pressing them into the floor and stand tall. Inhale, and on the exhale lengthen forward and rest your hands on your thighs, shoulders relaxed down away from the ears. Inhale and exhale deeply, then hold the breath out. Holding the breath out, strongly draw the belly button in toward the spine and suck the abdomen upward, as if it were moving up under the ribcage. Hold the breath in for several heartbeats, then release, and inhale as you return to a standing position.

Stage 2: Repeat Stage 1 to the point where the abdomen is drawn in. Holding the breath out, pump the abdomen in and out several times. Exhale, release, and inhale up to standing. Repeat this three times.

If holding your breath is new to you, begin with short holdings and avoid straining.

Taking the additive approach

Most of us find it easier to add new healthy behaviors and habits than to drop unhealthy ones. By taking the tact of adding positive behaviors before removing negative behaviors, the sense of deprivation often accompanying behavior change may be attenuated. For example, often in the initial nutrition counseling session, it becomes clear that the individual takes fewer servings of fruits and vegetables than the national recommendations of five a day. This is an opportunity to have a goal of adding servings of fruits and vegetables as a first step to change. Then, some unhealthy foods may simply drop

"I have had my transformation!" said Anita toward the end of the workshop series. "I've got plenty to work on and I still stumble, but whoa, I've really been nudged along. This was just what I needed. You know, my doctor said to me, 'Anita, you need to lose at least 10% of your body weight.' Well, yeah! Does he think I like to weigh what I do? No one has ever really told me how to do it and hung in there with me through the obstacles. That's why I think gastric bypass looks so good to so many really overweight people—I'm so glad I found this other way!"

out of the diet, and the subtractive goals (e.g., to reduce overeating unhealthy foods) may seem less daunting. Can you think of ways to take an additive approach to change?

During the challenging transition of behaviors, a nutrition professional can guide you with realistic goal setting and help with self-monitoring and appropriate encouragement to keep you moving when you are ready to give up. During these periods, a nutrition professional may remind you that most individuals find the process difficult, and as you master new skills specific barriers will likely be overcome.

Below I've described how concepts and exercises discussed in this chapter may be incorporated into your personal program.

Sample Program for a Week: Exploring Change

- Review Diet Manifestation worksheet, and update as needed

- Negative Stress Cycle Exploration exercise

- Take a beginners' yoga class 1-2x/week
  or
  Follow a beginners' yoga CD/DVD practice 1-2x/week
  or
  Practice centering, cat and dog breathing warm-up, stomach-pumping breath, salutation to the sun (begin with 2 or 3 repetitions, and increase to 10 repetitions), relaxation

- Change Boosters exercise

- Review and update goals, if necessary

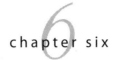
balance: an east-west view of moderation

Contradictions have always existed in the soul of man. But it is only when we prefer analysis to silence that they become a constant and insoluble problem. We are not meant to resolve all contradictions but to live with them and rise above them.

— WILLIAM BLAKE

What Is Moderation?

In order to lead a happy and productive life everyone needs moderation, and we all know when we don't have it. But just what is moderation, and how can you be moderate in an anything-but-moderate world?

A moderate lifestyle is a healthy one. Many of us can reel off the basics of a moderate lifestyle: generally sticking to an eating plan rich in fruit, vegetables, whole grains, and lean proteins, and general adherence to the "Guidelines for Americans," which includes things like maintaining a healthy weight, avoiding too much sugar and salt, and

Tom said, "You know, my doctor tells me every time I see him that I need to lose weight. But we never do talk about just how to do that. So I never took the first step until now. I've had the gastric bypass talk, too, and while it may work and I know people's lives have really been saved by it, it's major surgery…I want to try other things first. Like moderation! I definitely need a moderation coach."

working with a nutrition professional if your weight or other medical condition necessitates lifestyle change.

As we've seen, physical activity is another anchor of a moderate lifestyle. National fitness organizations recommend we be more physically active than most of us really are. Definitions and examples of a moderate lifestyle are clear and widely available, but the majority of Americans can't seem to incorporate concepts of moderation into our daily lives. Cultural norms present moderation as passive, a little boring, and even undesirable, as exaggerated by Oscar Wilde's famous observations: "Moderation is a fatal thing" and "Nothing succeeds like excess."

Yogic Moderation: Standing in the Fire

Yoga's philosophical framework of the yamas and niyamas richly and clearly describe the mental framework of a moderate approach to lifestyle. While national health recommendations provide general outlines as to what a moderate lifestyle is, the actual how-to is much harder to find. In yoga, moderation is not a passive state easily achieved. The moderate yoga practitioner is a spiritual warrior constantly challenged by his or her own attachments (things he or she is drawn to, appetites) and aversions (things he or she pushes away from, dislikes). If the practitioner can

"No question I'm attached to my pattern. It's great at the end of the day to slide into my chair with a beer and watch TV," said Tom. "Very attached. I'm tired then, too, so that feeds into my being resistant, or inert, to doing much else."

begin to attenuate his or her appetites and dislikes through following the yamas and niyamas, and direct his or her passion (tapas) toward self-study (svadhyaya) or self-care, a more moderate lifestyle may be achieved, and his or her spiritual journey will proceed unencumbered. This cognitive restructuring, the re-weaving of your thinking process, is a difficult undertaking. In yoga it is sometimes referred to as "standing in the fire" between the two poles of attachment and aversion.

"Speaking of aversions, I think most men think yoga is for women," said Tom. "I knew the stretching would be good for me, but I've found that I'm definitely getting a cardio workout in the more active classes. Yoga is definitely not for wimps! I care less about that perception, too, as my body and my head feel so good after it."

Modern yoga culture itself, however, is not immune to duplicity. With the tremendous gain in popularity of the practice and resultant explosion of commercial yoga endeavors, there is a booming yoga media culture that implies that if you purchase certain yoga products you will easily find unending bliss, happiness, and a perfect yoga butt. In these image-pitches there is no hint of the hours of sadhana (practice) or the years of self-development necessary for the average practitioner to reach the states of bliss and physical perfection being peddled. This body-ism of getting overly attached to our physical appearance is prevalent in the yoga world, but it is simply another distraction blocking your path to becoming a fully aware human.

"I've always liked 'follow your bliss' as a life motto, though I've struggled to do that," said Barbara. "When I first heard of yoga's balance concept, I wondered how I could follow my bliss and be unattached. But as I consider it in my life, it makes more sense. Sometimes you can get so wrapped up in following your bliss that it's just all about a short-term charge. Combining these two philosophies works for me. I try to do things I enjoy, but remember not to get too attached to any one thing. It does make me feel more balanced to take life that way."

> "I've always been an emotion ignorer," said Tom. "And tempers can get hot in my business. Annie suggested I add little walks into my workday—just a 5-minute around-the-block thing. I do it when things get too intense or just make sure to take two or three through the day and it really does help. Just to move and decompress through the day."

Enjoy your fit body, your vibrant energy, but remember not to take it too seriously. The journey is the practice, and there is no goal or destination other than being in the present moment in practice and in life. You are already there, perfect in your imperfections, regardless of your brand of yoga pants.

Dynamic Stability: Integrating Strong Emotions

In your exploration of moderation, a professional may assist you in learning to ride the emotional cycles of unconscious reactions to life events that may negatively impact your long-term health. Many eating disorders and unhealthy behaviors are born of the need to integrate strong emotions. One yoga-based model to do this, developed by counselor and yogini Sandra Scherer (Dayashakti), is called The Wave Work®. In this model, when an incident occurs you remain fully conscious and attentive to your emotions without avoiding or curtailing the experience. According to Scherer, emotions have a natural cycle of peaking and receding. If you "ride the wave" of your emotions, they will be expressed rather than repressed. Repressed emotion has a way of sneaking back later to be expressed in unhealthy ways. Here's an example: Imagine a small child, whom you may see tumbling through these waves several times in the course of an hour. Say the child falls and gets a small bump on his head, more a scare than an injury. After a momentary pause, when the child recovers from his initial confusion and realizes that his head hurts, he bursts into tears.

This is the point at which many parents say, "Oh, don't cry, you are not hurt badly," encouraging the child to regain his composure as quickly as possible. If the parent allows the child to "ride the wave," he or she may say something more akin to, "That must have hurt. I'm right here for you." According to the theory, there will be a point at which the child's cries naturally subside and he moves on with the experience integrated and less likely to come back to haunt him later. The process of "riding the wave of emotion" is illustrated in Chart 14. You can find out where to learn more about The Wave Work® in the Resources for Further Study section.

This process may be used to help you integrate strong emotions, to work with both sensation and emotion in your yoga practice, to explore the roots of emotional eating, and to work with your emotions in everyday life.

"I've been riding the wave in my yoga practice," said Christine. "The other day, in a yoga posture a familiar emotion of being embarrassed about my body came over me. Rather than my usual way of moving on to other thoughts, I held the emotion and tried to observe how it felt, physically, mentally, and at an "energetic" level. It was definitely not comfortable but I stayed with it, I continued to examine the emotion, hold my yoga posture, breathe steadily, and relax, and something shifted. In my mind, I clearly saw my first boyfriend, who used to make nasty comments about my soft belly and arms. I really hated that but haven't thought much about it. I see now that my embarrassment is a choice I'm making—to hang on to an insensitive comment that someone made to me a long time ago—and I can make the choice to feel differently about my body now. All that, in a yoga posture!"

Chart 14: Riding the Wave of Emotion or Sensation

The practice of being present for experience:

❧ Watch   ❧ Feel   ❧ Allow

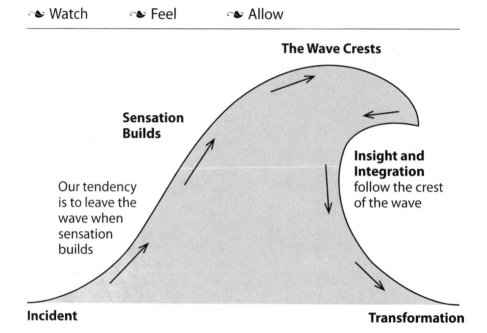

The Wave Crests

**Sensation
Builds**

**Insight and
Integration**
follow the crest
of the wave

Our tendency
is to leave the
wave when
sensation
builds

Incident   **Transformation**

Source: The Wave Work Fellowship. The Wave Work®. Accessed at www.wavework.com. June 2006.

Yoga and Meditation Tools for Exploring Balance and Moderation

Exercises 20–23 include journaling and physical exercises that may help you develop the valuable skill of balancing. There are a few universal principles to balancing, helpful in yoga poses and in life. These include:

❧ Focus your gaze (called drishti in yoga) at something that is not going to move. A point on the floor or wall works. A person in front of you—not so good. He or she will inevitably bobble.

⟳ Grow your roots. Lift and fan your toes so that your feet are wide and stable, and imagine your roots reaching far into the earth beneath you. Remember the old Batman series where the room would tilt? No problem for you, you've got your big wide lotus feet growing roots to anchor you.

⟳ Keep both your gaze and your breath steady and soft. As an experiment, you can dart your eyes around the room and see if that destabilizes you. The same thing may happen if you try rapid breathing. Anchor the breath. Anchor the drishti. Root down, so that your trunk and limbs can reach to the sky. Notice if you are clenching your jaw or tightening other parts of your body.

Exercise 20: Journaling: Satya (Truthfulness)

Find a quiet place to journal. The questions in this exercise may activate deep feelings. If that happens, stay relaxed, breathe, and either examine or simply observe your emotion and how it physically feels in your body, consciously allowing your heart to melt out of compassion for yourself. With continued practice, cultivating calm abiding, this process can help you integrate these feelings into the full reality of who you are.

Truthfulness (satya): We all know how challenging it can be to live in truth. But, by increasing awareness of satya, we can harvest the life energy that we waste in avoiding the truth, for use in powering our life's true journey.

1) Are you honest with yourself with regards to the amount of food you eat? The amount of physical activity you get?

2) When you make resolutions around your weight and eating, do you make them in a way that cannot be achieved, or without making the preparations to support the resolution? Can you

set an intention that is both compassionate and achievable—a goal you are more than 80% sure you can attain? What might that be? What might you do in preparation to support your resolution?

3) Do you acknowledge and feel your full range of emotions? Neither suppressing "negative" emotions, nor clinging to "positive" feelings?

4) What are the messages your mind chatters about—your self-talk? Are you aware of when you are judging yourself or others? When your ego is talking? Can you see "both/and" qualities, as opposed to "either/or" propositions?

5) Do you really believe you are divine? Have you gotten glimpses of that feeling? Journal about how you feel about yourself on the deepest level you can access right now. Keep working to drop deeper.

Exercise 21: Balancing: Tree (Vrksasana)

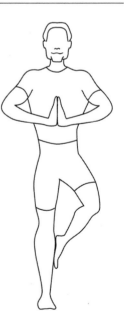

Benefits: Aids balance and concentration.

Contraindications: None, if modifications are done for knee or balance requirements.

Here is what vrksasana may look like:

Instructions: Stand tall in tadasana, roots of the big toes touching and legs active. Engage the abdomen and reach the crown of your head upward. Focus your gaze on a fixed point. Softly anchor your drishti on this point. Press your hands together in prayer position in front of the heart. Shift your weight to your right leg. Feel the foot rooted into the floor, the leg strong like the trunk of a tree. Then, lift your left foot off the floor and place the sole of the foot either on the inner right ankle, calf, or groin, depending on which is accessible and comfortable. Press the left foot gently into the right leg, and press the leg gently back into the foot, like an embracing. Lengthen again through the crown of the head, feeling the heart lift and keeping the abdomen strong. If you feel steady, let your hands reach overhead, either joining them in prayer position over your head or keeping them shoulder-width apart. Reach upward through the fingers. Inhale, and on the exhale release the palms back to prayer position in front of the heart, and release the left foot to the floor. Repeat on the other side.

Modification: If this standing balance posture is difficult for you, begin standing with your back to a wall for support, and do the posture from there. Be patient and cultivate steadiness.

Exercise 22: Balancing and Core Strength (Navasana)

Benefits: Strengthens abdomen and back. Aids concentration.

Contraindications: Recent abdominal surgery. If the back is weak, prevent strain by beginning in the easier stage of the posture and proceed slowly as strength increases.

Here are what Stages 1 and 3 may look like:

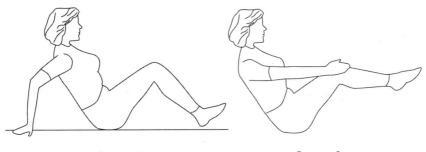

Stage 1   Stage 3

Instructions:

Stage 1: Sit on your mat with your legs out in front of you. Bend your knees and place your feet flat on the floor, hip-width apart. Sit up straight, and activate the abdomen by drawing the belly button in toward the spine. Reach your hands a foot or so behind your hips, resting your fingertips on the floor. Engage the belly again; imagine there is a hand pressing firmly into the low back, and lift through the center of the chest so that the central core of your torso is very active. Feeling the press on your back and engaging your belly, lift your feet slightly off the floor. Breathe. Keep the chest light and lifting and the low back long by lifting up through the heart. Keep the abdomen strong. Breathe and lift the heart. Inhale, and on an exhale release the feet to the floor.

Stage 2: As in Stage 1, but lift the shins parallel to the floor. Keep the low back light and lifting and the abdomen and core engaged.

Stage 3: As in Stage 2, but reach the hands forward, parallel to the floor. Keep the shoulders releasing down and the spine long.

Stage 4: As in Stage 3, but begin to straighten the legs without compromising the back.

Throughout your practice of navasana, be conscious of sensations in the lower back. Remember not to strain. If you do feel strain, take an earlier stage of the posture, holding for a few extra breaths to strengthen the abdomen and core, before eventually moving to a deeper stage.

Exercise 23: Half Headstand (Ardha Sirsasana)

Benefits: Strengthens upper body and core. Getting upside down facilitates the cleansing aspects of our physiology. The exhale of the breath, which clears the lungs, is facilitated in inversion, venous return (especially when in full headstand) of blood to the heart is facilitated, as well as digestive elimination. Improves balance and concentration. Inversions often provide us practice for working with fear.

Contraindications: Those with uncontrolled glaucoma, uncontrolled hypertension, recent neck, back, or abdominal injury or surgery, or shoulder injury. Those with larger, rounder bodies may want to take particular care in working half headstand to avoid placing undue weight on the head and neck until the abdomen, core, and upper body have the strength and consciousness to support that weight. This is an excellent posture to learn under the guidance of a skilled teacher.

Here's what this posture may look like as you reach Stage 2 or 3:

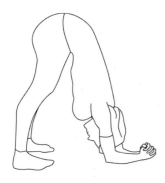

Instructions:

Stage 1: Begin in a table position with the palms down, directly under the shoulders. Sit the hips back and exhale down onto the elbows. The elbows will be shoulder-width apart (or less than shoulder-width if you have flexible shoulders). Drag the hands together and intertwine your fingers. Notice that there is one pinky finger at the bottom of your intertwined hands; tuck that finger into the palm so that it is in line with the opposite pinky and the edges of the outer palm and the outer wrist are flat on the floor. Take a look at your wrists and see that they neither collapse in nor roll out, but are straight (think of making a karate chop—nice straight wrists). Rest your head between your hands, the very crown of the head just kissing the floor. Press into your forearms and lift your head off the floor, so the neck can be long. Your forearms descend into the floor, and the shoulders lift away from the floor. This is a primary action of a headstand—to lift the shoulders and lengthen the neck. Think of keeping the shoulders over the elbows and the armpit inflated, so the base of your posture is strong and stable. Bring the crown of the head back to the floor, and see if you can get the same lift through the shoulders and lengthening of the neck without lifting your head off the floor. Invite the shoulders out over the elbows, and if your elbows slide out wider than your shoulders, come down, reposition, and try again.

Stage 2: Now roll your toes under (so the balls of your feet are on the floor, toes stretching forward) and lift your hips toward the sky as in downward-facing dog, knees soft. Again, let the crown of the head touch-kiss the floor between the hands/wrists. Engage the abdomen and core by drawing the belly button in toward the spine. Activate the shoulders by pressing into the forearms and lifting the head off the floor, keeping the neck long, allowing the engagement of the core to lift the shoulders. Place the crown of the head back down, but keep the lifting sensation in the shoulders and the engagement of the belly and core. Work for several breaths, then rest in child's pose by drawing the hips back to rest on the heels, letting the forehead rest on the floor.

Stage 3: Repeat Stage 2, and as you gain strength, begin to walk your toes in, lifting your hips until they eventually come over the shoulders. Keep the upper back long, shoulders lifting, base of the posture strong and abdomen engaged. It may be easier to envision coming into a full headstand once you feel the lift from the belly and the hips are over the shoulders. Proceed slowly and remember to keep the integrity of the base of the posture—elbows under shoulders, neck long, shoulders lifting.

Stage 4: Work in Stage 3, and then lift one leg up, keeping the base of the posture steady. Activate the core, flex into the feet, and slowly lift the other leg overhead. Remember to keep the neck long and the forearms descending. As you gain skill in this posture, you may try lifting the legs together, which is a greater challenge, but ensure that you are using your abdomen. Let your sirsasana be a long-term project. There is no need to race into the posture until you develop the strength and awareness to do it with conscious intelligence.

 "Thinking of doing a headstand really freaked me out. Doing the standing balances was challenging for me, so what am I doing trying a half headstand? But Annie has helped me get the alignment right, and the stronger I get, the more often I think maybe someday I will stand on my head," said Tom. "I don't even know if I ever want to stand on my head, but I like where the exercise takes me...opens up my eyes a little wider. It's fun to get upside down!"

Sample Program for a Week: Exploring Balance

- Review goals and affirmations, and update as needed

- Review exercises from Chapters Four through Six, and repeat those that were helpful

- Chapter Six journaling exercise

- Take a beginners' yoga class
  or
  Follow a beginners' yoga CD/DVD 1-2x/week
  or
  Practice centering, warm-ups including cat and dog breathing, stomach-pumping breath, salutation to the sun, tree, core strength, half headstand, relaxation

connection: relationship and renewal

Our deepest fear is not that we are inadequate.
Our deepest fear is that we are powerful beyond measure.

We ask ourselves, who am I to be brilliant, gorgeous,
talented and fabulous? Actually who are you not to be?

...as we let our own light shine, we unconsciously give other
people permission to do the same. As we are liberated from
our own fear, our presence automatically liberates others.

— MARIANNE WILLIAMSON

Relationships in Physical and Emotional Health

Why do some people who seem to do "all the right things" still get struck with chronic conditions such as cancer? Why is living to age 100 free of chronic disease not unusual in some rural traditional cultures? A number of large studies have compared diet, stress levels, culture, and life expectancy among various peoples of the world. We are learning more every day about the subtle aspects of our modern culture that tend to make us sick. But research is just beginning to

"I have a great life, but the busy-ness is getting to me," said Suzanne. "And relationships just don't seem as easy as they once were. I have a difficult relationship with my mother, who can be critical and downright nasty. No question it increases my stress level, and now that she's ill, I see her all the time. Of course I can't cut off my relationship with her—she's not a real threat to my well-being and I love her. I've tried not to let her tirades impact me so much, but haven't been able to do that. All my family relationships feel the ripple of when she's really tough. My relationships with my husband and my daughter get a little more strained then too."

evaluate how social support (the quality and number of relationships you have) impacts your long-term health. Interesting early findings suggest that stable social support may decrease hospitalizations, help you recover from disease, and improve chronic low back pain. And the discoveries (and rediscoveries) are just beginning.

You are your relationships. Family, work, community, and interpersonal relationships are a medium through which you express yourself in society. Your relationships reflect your early conditioning, conscious desires, and unconscious psychological landscape. Relationships require ongoing choices. When someone with alcoholism goes through a 12-step program, he or she examines his or her relationships to determine which are supportive of a sober life and which are not. If you make major transitions to a healthy lifestyle, or if you lose a large amount of weight, you in essence become another person, or at the very least another version of yourself. During a major life transition, a 12-step style inventory of your past and your

"Oh, I definitely have friends who don't support my healthy lifestyle, but it makes me really sad to think of just cutting them out of my life," said Christine. "Some of my unhealthy friends are so fun to be around! I guess I can think about just how these friends impact me, health-wise, and if there are ways I can be with them and stay the course. The restaurant scene is definitely a challenge."

relationships may help your transformation stick. Several resources that can help you learn more about this style of inventory are listed in the Resources for Further Study section of this book.

What is a healthy relationship?

All healthy relationships ebb and flow. There are times that we're angry at or tired of even our dearest friends and family. And even in apparently simple communication, humans have the capacity for chasms of misunderstanding. As many Eastern teachers describe, relationships provide wonderful ongoing practice for softening your heart. When someone disappoints or misunderstands or lashes out or worse, can you soften and open your heart to him or her and to yourself in the situation?

"I can see how yoga philosophy can help me take a step back in the heat of a clash with my mom," Suzanne said. By trying to take care of myself and be as compassionate to her as I can be, I can just work all that emotion that's swelled up. Simple, but not easy!"*

Yoga philosophy offers guidance for relationships in the yamas and niyamas. The yamas, which include ahimsa (non-violence), satya (truthfulness), asteya (non-stealing), brahmacharya (continence or control of the life force), and aparigraha (non-coveting, generosity), are yoga's guidelines governing societal and personal relationships. Yamas also pertain to your self-care relationship. Healthy relationships are rich in the qualities described in the yamas.

Niyamas are observances that focus primarily on your relationship with your own physical, intellectual, emotional, energetic, and spiritual selves. The niyamas include saucha (purity, cleanliness), santosa (contentment), tapas (passion or heat), svadhyaya (self-study), and Isvara pranidhana (dedication to a greater power, or connection to God). Yogis often teach that yoga practice is to a great extent about examining and improving relationships with others, ourselves, and

What is a healthy relationship?

According to psychologists and health educators at Columbia University, a healthy relationship is when:

- You disagree and you know it's OK to talk about your differences.
- You make decisions together.
- You listen to each other's viewpoints and feelings.
- You negotiate when you have conflict and find a mutually satisfactory way to compromise.
- You feel comfortable taking time alone if you need it and feel alright doing some things separately.
- There's no fear in your relationship.
- You don't restrict or control each other.
- You respect and value each other.

the divine. As your practice develops, your relationships will likewise develop through your practice of the yamas and niyamas. As that happens, you will proceed along your journey toward becoming your fullest realized you. This journey may also be described as moving through the eight-limbed path of yoga. The eight-limbed path and the yamas and niyamas were discussed in detail in Chapter Two.

Here is a wonderful meditation, and an exercise to help you explore your inner connection. Yogis call this meditation different things, from "meditation in motion" to "authentic movement" to "free flowing with prana." There isn't a diagram or picture to show you how to do it. It is simply learning to hear that quiet voice inside and following it through physical movement.

Exercise 24: Moving Meditation

Benefits: Excellent practice for developing the ability to move with the breath and to differentiate between when you are moving from a place of authenticity and when you are moving in response to external directives.

Contraindications: None, except to honor your physical limitations.

Instructions: Set up your yoga space, or find an area that you can move freely in. For the first few times you do this, it may be helpful to use light, flowing music if you have it. If not, the sound of your breath should suffice.

Stand at the top of your mat. Close your eyes and find the thread of your breath. Begin to invite your body into its yogic alignment; root into the feet, feel the heart lift, open the ears, and let breath help you create internal space. When you feel compelled to move, slowly begin a sun salutation. Move slowly, and whatever speed you are moving, see if you can cut it in half. Slow way down. Feel the breath move inside as you slow your physical movements way down. Then, staying connected to your breath and the prana it holds, see if you can feel the urge to move in another way, beyond the sun salutation. Keep reconnecting with the breath, and simply begin to allow your breath and prana to move you. You may find that you are moving along and focusing deep, then sort of wake up or pull out of the meditative movement. If that happens, slow down again or stop, and focus on the breath until you feel compelled to move again. It's almost as if you sit back and watch yourself flow. It doesn't have to look like anything in particular. Just flow with attunement to your own breath, and focus on the sensation in your body.

You can free-flow for several minutes, and then stop in a yoga posture. Then, you can flow again, or rest in savasana.

Exercise 25: Internal Relationship Meditation

Benefits: Aids shift in self-regard.

Contraindications: If it is not comfortable to lie on your back, find another comfortable resting position, possibly with the aid of cushions or other props.

Instructions: Find a comfortable place to lie down on your back, face up. You might place a cushion or blanket under your knees or make other adjustments so that your low back can relax and you are able to lie quietly for about 10 minutes. Let your palms face up toward the ceiling, hands 4-5 inches from the body. Let the legs relax, feet falling to the side. Feel the whole body resting on the floor, heavy and relaxed. Listen to your relaxed body inhale and exhale for 10-12 breaths.

Begin to imagine yourself floating near the ceiling, looking down at your body. Rather than seeing this body as yours, imagine that it is your dearest friend, or perhaps a brother or sister. Are you able to be more compassionate toward this person? Do you have good wishes or intentions to send him or her? Can you see the external and internal beauty of this person? Do you have anything to tell him or her? Take time to observe and to relate to this beloved person. When you are finished, begin to deepen your breath, and slowly wiggle your fingers and toes. When you are ready, roll to one side, and press yourself up to a comfortable seated position. It may be valuable to journal about any thoughts or insights you experienced during this exercise.

Developing Communities of Support

Positive change doesn't happen in a vacuum. As you examine and improve your lifestyle, a network of likeminded individuals is critical to support your lasting maintenance.

How do you develop a healthy relationship?

- ∿ By being honest with each other.
- ∿ By giving each other room to breathe.
- ∿ By being responsible for your own feelings and valuing yourself.
- ∿ By not expecting the other person to solve all your problems or give you everything you are going to need.
- ∿ By telling the truth even when it's difficult ... not to hurt feelings, but to respect yourself and others you care about.
- ∿ By getting rid of any chip on your shoulder.
- ∿ By not letting anyone treat you like a doormat.
- ∿ By treating someone as you would like to be treated.

The cultivation of healthy relationships and social supports necessitates that you access a higher-than-normal state of consciousness (witness consciousness), looking beyond your individual needs and desires to a more global way of thinking. As discussed in Chapter Two, the practice of meditation allows you to more easily move between various states of consciousness, and particularly to access a global or higher consciousness. Ironically, the solitary practice of meditation is conducive to healthy relationships as it helps you shift your perspective.

"Well, a lot of the tips for how to develop a healthy relationship just may not happen with Mom. But to me, it's really how I respond," said Suzanne. "This is all great training for my real estate work. Lots of revved-up relationships there, too. Lots of opportunities to practice yamas and niyamas."

Building a supportive community of likeminded individuals is an ongoing process that takes time and effort. Even just a few connections may provide the support you need to continually adjust to lifestyle changes. Yoga classes, fitness classes, meetings such as Weight Watchers or Overeaters Anonymous, churches, and community events are all places where you may find likeminded people. The ability to connect with others at gatherings is a skill that improves with practice. The Internet also provides connections to countless forums, listservs, and opportunities to connect with others, although some studies suggest that the quality of face-to-face contact seems to provide the best sense of connectedness. Your social network will be as individual as you are, and can provide you a sounding board and opportunities to assist and be assisted by others in making changes or adhering to a healthy lifestyle.

One connecting activity to do with someone else is partner yoga. Another person's body is the ultimate yoga prop. It's moldable, has weight, breathes, and giggles. Partner yoga postures explore the yoga of a physical contact relationship. You can get a great stretch working with a partner, have an opportunity to explore the experience of another's breath up close, and have fun. Here are several partner yoga postures to try with a friend.

> "You know, I haven't had support like this yoga workshop group in a long time, if ever," said Suzanne. "I realize that so much of my social world has to do with work. But this is just for me. In this group we're sharing our problems but also working together to really do something about them. I love this group of people, and I really care about their progress. It's a great support group that I think will help us all out from here on in."

Exercise 26: Partner Yoga Postures: Simple Partner Breathing

Benefits: Provides a safe context to explore aspects of relationships

Contraindications: None.

Here's how the inhale of this posture may look:

Instructions: Find a partner of similar size. Stand facing each other, about 18 inches apart. Let the feet be directly under the hips. Root your feet into the floor, and both partners bring arms out to a T position. Let your palms come together, and adjust the distance between you so that you are physically comfortable. Close your eyes, and on an inhale, keeping your palms on your partner's, lift your arms overhead. Continue to stay in contact as you exhale your arms back down toward your sides. Inhale up and exhale down several times. Do you need to communicate with your partner? How do you do that? Does this exercise bring you more in sync with your partner? Can you sense how each of you is adjusting to and influencing the other? Exhale, bringing your arms down, and bow to each other in thanks.

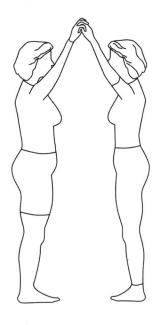

Exercise 27: Partner Seated Twist

Benefits: Aids exploration of relationships, promotes lengthening and freeing of the spine, massages the internal organs (possibly promoting digestion).

Modifications: A strap may be necessary for those who are less flexible or have a larger body. If sitting cross-legged on the floor is very uncomfortable, even with the aid of blankets under the sacrum, a solo spinal twist in a chair may substitute.

Here is how this partner posture may look:

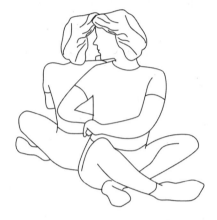

Instructions: Sit cross-legged on the floor, facing away from your partner, resting your back on each other's. Both partners reach the right arm out to the side as you relax your right shoulder down away from your right ear.

Bend the right elbow and wrap your right arm behind your back. Reach your left hand forward and across to the right so that you can reach around and take your partner's right hand behind his or her back (use a strap here if needed). Sit up straight with both hands clasping your partner's, making any adjustments needed for comfort. On an inhale extend through the crown of your head, rooting down through the sitz bones at the base of your spine. On the exhale, let the spine twist around to the right in a smooth, relaxed way. Inhale, extend, and exhale, deepening the twist as comfort allows. Let your eyes complete the twist, and imagine that you are looking to the past, to the life that you have led to this date. Communicate with your partner to either deepen the twist or ease off. Work for 5-6 breaths, and slowly unwind. Repeat on the other side. Once you are in the twist on the second side, finish the twist with the movement of the eyes, and imagine that you are looking at your life from this point forward. Work for several more breaths and release. Face your partner. Place your right hand over her heart, and your left hand on top of hers. Acknowledge her role in your journey (if you can), and wish her well on hers. Bow in thanks, and release.

Detoxification for Physical and Emotional Health

When you reorganize a closet or a room, you identify and clear out the clothing or items you no longer want or need. Often once a closet is cleared out, you feel that your whole wardrobe has improved. Likewise, in the process of changing habits, you occasionally need to clean house. Do you have habits, beliefs, and relationships that no longer aid your growth? What would it take to clear or modify them, making way for new, more conscious paradigms to take hold?

In the past decades, detoxification has gone from an area rife with dietary fads and fraud to one of exciting discoveries. There is a growing body of research examining the role of nutrition in aiding the body with the clearing of toxic substances. In 2002, the Environmental Protection Agency (EPA) estimated that 4,793 billion pounds of chemical pollutants were released into the environment in the United States, which is more than 16 pounds for every American! Researchers argue that while the body is designed to clear toxins, the large toxic load we ingest often leads to health problems such as headaches, muscle and joint pain, chronic fatigue, and allergy- or flu-like symptoms. Nutritional detoxification may be helpful to you in using yoga and meditation as tools for weight management. If you happen to have any of the symptoms outlined above, if you tend to eat a highly refined diet, have a high-stress lifestyle, or are exposed to a toxic environment, you may benefit from detoxification. Nutritional detox programs range from short, several-day elimination diets consisting of fruits and vegetables and avoiding caffeine, red meat, dairy, soda, or other foods to longer, supplemented, "supported" fasts. A gentle detoxification period with special attention to diet may give you a psychological boost as you undergo lifestyle changes, effectively marking your transition to healthier eating. If you tend to struggle with compulsive eating or are drawn toward fad diets, however, you may not be a good candidate for detoxification programs. If normal healthy eating is a huge step for you, then occasional detoxification may just confuse or complicate your ability to remain focused on daily healthy eating and daily lifestyle behaviors. It's the everyday habits that will make the real difference in your life, not the occasional detox.

Nutritional detoxification remains controversial, in part because some of the most well-known researchers in this area also promote their own brands of nutrition supplements directly to the consumers they advise, which the AMA (American Medical Association) and the ADA (American Dietetic Association) identify as a potentially unethical conflict of interest. Ethically, it can get complicated if a therapeutic relationship (built on confidences, trust, and your best medical interests) becomes entangled with a sales-marketing relationship (in which the salesperson persuades the consumer to purchase a product). If a professional gives you dietary advice, and that advice entails purchasing supplements from that professional, you need to be informed just how much money he or she is making from the supplements and if there are other products on the market you might also select. This is an area many therapists struggle with, and just because your therapist also sells supplements does not necessarily mean that he or

"You know, I've heard about detoxing, and it really appeals to me," said Suzanne. *"The more I learn about aging and about toxins, the more I think that detoxing is great for the aging person, so I will definitely check it out. I'm also in a business that can really be tough—not always, but at times people can be pretty horrible to each other. I could detox from that a little too!"*

"I think that you'd really benefit, too, from beginning with detoxing that took you out of your busy life. Maybe go to a spa or retreat," I said. "Then you could begin to take the best of what worked for you in the relaxing spa life, and begin to work it into your regular life. Remember, the best detox is a clean diet and healthy moderate lifestyle on most days, if not every day."

she is unethical…it's just a very grey area. Despite the ethical muddiness, nutritional detoxification remains an exciting area of nutrition research and practice. For a safe and effective detoxification regimen, it's best if you have a full nutritional assessment, careful individualized design of your program, and close follow-up. So working with a nutrition professional is an excellent idea. Safe and gentle nutritional detoxification may be synergistic with a yoga and meditation practice. Because detoxification regimens are highly individualized, specific recommendations are beyond the scope of this book. References for further investigation are provided in the Resources for Further Study section.

"I'm drawn to detoxing too, but I know that part of its appeal is the same thing that draws me to the binge-purge," said Christine. "So, someday it may be good for me, but for right now, I'll focus on just eating an overall healthy diet and following a healthy lifestyle most of the time… steadiness."

Nutritional detox is not the only detox you can do. How about a media fast—with no cell phone, email, Internet, radio, or TV? A clutter detoxification of your home or office? How about a relationship detox, wherein you take one relationship and journal about it, using the yamas and niyamas as your guide? What can you clear? What can you simplify? There are a great variety of yogic detoxifications, from pranayama breathing exercises to most of the physical asanas, to other cleansing practices that are best suited for advanced practitioners. In yoga energetics, the legs and hips are the conduit between the universal energy source of the earth and the higher centers of the human body, being the belly (hara), heart, head, and crown. When you work to open your hips, you clear the channels to your higher centers. Some yogis say that strong emotions we block can get snagged in the hips, so if you hold a hip opener for some time, you may feel waves of strong emotion. Just breathe, relax, allow, and feel the wave of emotion wash over you. This is the practice of integrating samskara. Here's a deep hip opener to add to your practice.

Exercise 28: Half Pigeon Pose (Ardha Kapotasana)

Benefits: Stretches and opens the hips, stretches the low back. Some yogis say that unresolved emotion often gets caught in the hips, causing tension; practicing hip openers helps to release that tension, allowing a clearer, stronger connection to the ground and allowing the practitioner to more efficiently draw energy from the earth.

Contraindications: Recent or severe knee injury or surgery, back surgery, or severe back problems. If you have knee problems, take this very gently.

Here is how this posture may look:

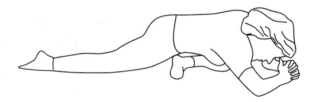

Instructions: Come to your hands and knees in a table position. Place a cushion to your right. Draw your right knee forward and between your hands (if you know your hips are tight), or outside of your right hand (if you have more flexibility in your hips), and bring the cushion under your right hip, so that you can sit back onto it. Flex your right foot. Let the left leg extend behind you. Notice your forward knee, and if you feel any strain there, you might draw the knee toward the centerline of the body to reduce that. If your hips are very tight, you may end up with your knee straight ahead, sitting back nearly on your right heel or with a cushion under the hip. If your hips are very open and flexible, your knee will be out to the side, and you can increase the stretch in the hip by drawing the right shin toward the top of your mat and your right heel toward the midline of the body, aware all the while of any strain in the knee that can be triggered when opening the hip in this posture. Adjust yourself to keep the stretch in the right hip and strain out of the right knee. Notice your back leg. Let it be straight, big toe and little toes pressing into the floor. Inhale and sit up and straight as the hips sink into the floor. On an exhale, slowly fold forward if you can, resting on your elbows or on a prop, and, as you become more flexible, allowing your forehead to drop toward the floor. Breathe into and relax the right hip, and breathe space into the right hip socket. Avoid pushing into the hip; just relax it and allow it to release. Breathe here for 5-6 breaths, and then slowly make your way back to a table position. Repeat on the other side.

The Spice of Challenge and Self-Study

Yoga provides infinite possibilities for deeper study. With the explosive popularity of the practice over the last few decades, there are also more opportunities for advanced practice led by competent teachers. The yoga sequences in this book are appropriate for a first-time or beginning student. Each posture presented is the first of many progressively deeper versions requiring greater strength, flexibility, or concentration. If you are a more advanced yoga practitioner, the concepts in this program may be adapted to your more advanced asana practice.

With its emphasis on balance, concentration, and skillful use of breath, yoga is a discipline that can benefit you long into your senior years. And even if you consider yourself "athletically challenged," you will probably find areas of gratifying natural ability in your yoga practice. Finding a competent and compassionate teacher attentive to your limitations and abilities is an important ingredient for deeper development, particularly if you have a rounder body or are sedentary. There are excellent teachers out there! If you don't find one right away, please don't give up—they are out there.

If you struggle with negative body image, the practice of svadhyaya (self-study) may be particularly challenging but it can also be your treasure. To begin to develop compassion for yourself, to honor and respect your own body, to appreciate that your present life situation is a result of both unique physical and emotional experiences and an opportunity for personal growth, is an extremely challenging mindset to maintain. Let your yoga teach you to be fully present to all experiences, both the happy, blissful ones of life as well as the painful, challenging experiences. Here are some questions to aid your svadhyaya.

Exercise 29: Journaling: Asteya (Non-stealing), Aparigraha (Generosity, Non-hoarding), Brahmacharya (Continence, Control of the Life Force), Santosa (Contentment)

Benefits: Stress management, aids behavior change.

Contraindications: None.

Instructions: Prepare to journal by finding a comfortable, quiet place. Take a moment to quiet and center yourself.

Brahmacharya (continence, control of the life force)

1) Do you have relationships that come from an inner sense of incompleteness? How about relationships that come from a sense of mutual respect and celebration of your fullest self? (This may be the same relationship at different times...plenty to explore here.)

Aparigraha (generosity, non-hoarding), Asteya (non-stealing)

Living a healthy life in today's culture is an act of simplicity and renunciation.

2) Do you have food cravings? Nearly everyone does and there are various physiological and emotional imbalances underlying them. Do you know or can you intuit what they are? Does eating a balanced diet and being regularly physically active help to alleviate them?

3) Can you differentiate the motivations in your life that are external (such as financial success or social acceptance) and those that are internal (your passions or health)?

4) Can you recognize media and societal messages that appeal to your external motivations and foster unhappiness or desire? What might you do to negate them when encountering these messages? How might witness consciousness be helpful here?

Santosa (contentment)

5) Have you ever cultivated feeling content with life just as it is? Can you make that shift right now? (Practice, practice…this is a learned skill!)

Finding a Yoga Teacher, Finding a Therapist

For someone just beginning, or for continuing students of yoga, it is helpful to have professional instruction. Here are some questions that may help you find your first yoga teacher:

Questions to ask when choosing a yoga teacher:

- What type of yoga do you teach?
- Do you work with individuals with medical issues or special needs?
- How long have you been studying yoga?
- How long have you been teaching?
- Do you have students like me (e.g., unfit, overweight, disabled, or with other issues) in your classes?
- Do you do individual instruction?
- How much does that cost and what would I get out of that?

Should the nutrition practitioner or her client attend a yoga class and feel uncomfortable or unsafe, trying another teacher may be the best option. Like nutrition counseling, yoga practice is a highly personal endeavor, and yoga professionals understand that their students must feel safe and comfortable in order for the experience to be successful for all involved.

 "My yoga practice has become a friend. I love it!" said Suzanne. "And, the yoga clothes, I admit, appeal to the fashionista in me. I like that yoga is trendy. But to go deeper like this, really use it to balance the stress in my life, get some exercise, it really does the trick. I'm so glad I found it."

Following I've described how concepts and exercises discussed in this chapter may be incorporated into a client's personal program.

Sample Program for a Week: Exploring Relationships

- ❧ Review Diet Manifestation worksheet and goals, and update as needed

- ❧ Relationship journaling exercise

- ❧ Take a beginners' yoga class
  or
  Follow a beginners' yoga CD/DVD practice 1-2x/week
  or
  Practice centering, cat and dog breathing warm-up, stomach-pumping breath, salutation to the sun (begin with 2 or 3 repetitions, and increase to 10 repetitions), partner postures, half pigeon, relaxation

- ❧ Internal Relationship meditation

- ❧ Review and update goals, if necessary

epilogue

The teacher who walks in the shadow of the temple
among his followers, gives not of his wisdom
but rather of his faith and his lovingness.

If he is indeed wise he does not bid
you enter the house of his wisdom
but rather leads you to the threshold of your own mind.

— KAHLIL GIBRAN

The room was silent. Barbara, Tom, Suzanne, Anita, and Christine lay on their yoga mats with light blankets over them, pillows under their knees, and eye pillows in place. "Let your muscles soften, like butter on the counter on a warm day. Let your bones rest heavy on the floor," I said. "Just let go."

Barbara felt her breath expand softly within her chest. She had an image in her mind of a leaf floating on a stream, lightly traveling from her chest to her limbs, fingers, and toes. "I've never been this completely relaxed," she thought. "This is what letting go feels like." Then she drifted into deep, conscious relaxation.

Ten minutes later I invited the class to slowly awaken from their conscious yogic sleep (yoga nidra). They wiggled their fingers and toes, slowly rocked their heads, and rolled to one side. They gently pressed themselves up into a comfortable seated position.

We sat in silent meditation. "Focus on the breath," I said.

Barbara thought about how far she'd come in the 6 weeks the workshop had been meeting. She felt as though she had her life back and had a plan for taking care of herself even when her family and her job got frantic. She lost 5 pounds over the 6 weeks of workshops, and feels that the regular exercise she's been doing has changed her body for the better—more muscle, less fat. But her biggest shift is in her mind. She spends a lot more time dwelling on the good things about herself, and while she often hears her mind judging, she now recognizes it and stops it. So, she has more peace of mind.

Christine felt centered and happy. While her weight was the same as 6 weeks before, everything about the way she ate and thought about eating was different. She knew more about her eating disorder and knew the red flags that triggered it. She now deals with strong emotions by expressing them rather than eating. She cries more, yells a little more, but binge-purges quite a bit less. While releasing the need to be media-perfect is a long-term project for Christine, she sees the path she needs to follow to get there. For the first time in a long time, she likes who she is and how she looks.

Anita smiled. She thanked her body for being the container of her learning about how to take better care of herself. With so much unhealthy lifestyle history, Anita knows that she needs to stick with it for a while to see results. She also has a clearer idea of the high stakes her diagnosis of diabetes carries in terms of her health. She wants to be healthy and active as long as she can, so she has been just that for the last 5 weeks or so. Since paying attention to what she eats, walking at least a half hour each day, and doing a gentle yoga class twice a week, Anita has lost 5 pounds and feels energetic and optimistic.

Tom thought about how he felt like a different person than when he first walked into this room. "I've become a yogi," he chuckled to himself. "A meditating, fruit-eating yogi." He's really taken to the vigorous yoga, and by doing that along with watching what he eats and taking stress management walks, he's dropped over 10 pounds. The beer-TV thing has less appeal too, though once in a while he still does it and it feels great. But it's more a once-in-a-while special event than a nightly habit. Tom is still a guy's guy and is actually surfing and more active than he's been in years. And he still loves junk food and eats it on occasion, but he is more aware of how a particular choice might impact his health, and he's taking charge of those choices.

Suzanne opened her eyes a crack, peeking at the others in the room. "This has been such a great collection of people to go through this with," she thought. "I feel that I know them each so well. We're each so different, but we've all learned a little something about ourselves, and how to have a little fun and take better care of ourselves."

"Take a moment to bow to your own efforts, this afternoon, throughout the time we've spent together, and in your life," I said. "Let's join our voices and our energies together by chanting the sound of om."

The vibration of voices rolled around the room. Then again, the room fell into a peaceful silence. "Namaste," I said. "Namaste," they said as I bowed to each of them. "Namaste," they said as they bowed to each other and smiled.

learn more

Annie B. Kay delivers the inspiring strategies and techniques detailed in *Every Bite Is Divine* to individuals and organizations.

For information on speaking, workshops, personal or organizational consultation, contact Annie at: www.anniebkay.com.

Would you like to order additional copies of *Every Bite Is Divine* for friends?

At www.anniebkay.com, you can:

- Order *Every Bite Is Divine*
- Connect with others exploring whole health
- Sign up to receive Annie's free e-newsletter
- Find out where you can attend a workshop
- Tell us how we can support your healthy lifestyle
- And lots more

health professionals

Are you a nutrition professional, yoga teacher, or other health professional?

There are resources to help you blend *Every Bite Is Divine* principles into your practice.

You can find discussions specifically for yoga teachers and clinicians, and find out about workshops and other events at www. anniebkay.com.

You can also order *Yoga and Meditation: Tools for Weight Management*, a manual (164 pgs) that includes the scientific and clinical background for strategies presented in *Every Bite Is Divine*, and additional discussion and exercises designed to aid the nutrition professional in incorporating these powerful elements into his or her existing practice. Approved for 14 CPEUs by ADA (American Dietetic Association).

An order form is provided on the following page.

Yoga and Meditation: Tools for Weight Management by Annie Kay is published by Wolf Rinke Associates.

Order: "Yoga and Meditation:
Tools for Weight Management" CPEU program

Item #	Description	Qty	Price	Total
C175	Yoga and Meditation: Tools for Weight Management		$99.95	
	Additional Reporting Form (if sharing program)		$25.00	
	Subtotal from above			
	Shipping and Handling (table)			
	MD residents, add 5% sales tax			
	TOTAL			

Shipping & Handling:

$50 or less add $4.50

$51 to $100 add $7.00

$101 to $150 add $9.50

$151 to $200 add $12.00

$201 to $250 add $14.50

$251 to $300 add $17.00

$301 to $350 add $17.00

$351 to $400 add $22.00

Canada S&H x2

Foreign overseas S&H x4

Overnight shipping available—call for rates

Free Shipping on orders of $201 or more (USA Only)

Order online: http://www.wolfrinke.com/CEFILES/cenutr.html#C175

Or Fax: Your credit card order to (401) 531-9282

Or Call: (800) 828-9653

Or Mail to: Wolf Rinke Associates, Inc.
PO Box 350, Clarksville, MD 21029-0350

Payment

_____ Here is my check or Money Order for the TOTAL amount payable to Wolf Rinke Associates, Inc.

_____ Please charge $_____ to my

❏ Master Card   ❏ VISA   ❏ American Express   ❏ Discover

Credit Card #: _____

Expiration date: _____

Signature _____

(We need your cc#, the expiration date, and your signature to ship your charge order.)

> **100% Money-Back Guarantee, less shipping charges, within 90 days of purchase**

Please send my order to:

Name: _____

Telephone (daytime): _____

E-mail: _____

Circle your Association: ADA   DMA   AAFCS   ASFSA

Other: _____

Company: _____

Address: _____

City: _____

State: _____   Zip: _____

bibliography

Sources of Information Used in Every Bite Is Divine

Prologue

Barks, C., and J. Moyne. Translation. *The Essential Rumi*. New York: Harper Collins, 1995.

Introduction

Ramacharaka, Yogi. *Advanced Course in Yogi Philosophy and Oriental Occultism*. Chicago: The Yogi Publication Society, 1904.

Chapter One

American Psychiatric Association. *Practice Guidelines for Eating Disorders*. Washington, DC: American Psychiatric Press, 1992.

Coon, K., and K. Tucker. "Television and Children's Consumption Patterns: A Review of the Literature." *Minerva Pediatr* (Oct 2002).

Dingemans, A., M. Brun, and E. van Furth. "Binge Eating Disorder: A Review." *Int J Obes Relat Metab Disord* (Mar 2002).

Epel, E., B. McEwen, T. Seeman, K. Matthews, G. Castellazzo, K. D. Brownell, J. Bell, and J. R. Ickovics. "Stress and Body Shape: Stress-Induced Cortisol Secretion Is Consistently Greater Among Women with Central Fat." *Psychosom Med* (2000).

Griffin, J., and E. M. Berry. "A Modern-Day Holy Anorexia? Religious Language in Advertising and Anorexia Nervosa in the West." *Eur J Clin Nutr* (Jan 2003).

Hill Rice, V. *Handbook of Stress, Coping and Health*. Thousand Oaks, CA: Sage Publications, Inc, 2000.

Hoek, H., and D. van Hoeken. "Review of the Prevalence and Incidence of Eating Disorders." *Int J Eat Disord* (Dec 2003).

Kilbourn, J. *Killing Us Softly* [video]. Cambridge, MA: Cambridge Doc. Films, 1981.

Kilbourn, J. *Deadly Persuasion.* New York, NY: The Free Press, Simon & Schuster, 1999.

Malkin, A., K. Wornian, and J. Chrisler. "Women and Weight: Gender Messages on Magazine Covers." *Sex Roles: A Journal of Research* (Apr 1999).

Meneroff, C., R. Stein, N. Diehl, and K. Smilack. "From the Cleavers to the Clintons: Role Choices and Body Orientation as Reflected in Magazine Article Content." *Int J Eat Dis* 16 (1994): 167-76.

Miller, T., J. Coffman, and R. Linke. "Survey on Body Image, Weight and Diet of College Students." *J Am Diet Assoc* (1980).

Mokdad, A. H., B. A. Bowman, E. S. Ford, et al. "Prevalence of Obesity, Diabetes, and Obesity-Related Health Risk Factors." *JAMA* 289 (2003): 76–79.

National Center for Health Statistics. *Prevalence of Overweight and Obesity Among Adults, US 1999-2002.* Online. http://www.cdc.gov/nchs/products/pubs/pubd/hestats/obese/obse99.htm. Accessed May 2, 2006.

National Institutes of Health, National Cancer Institute. "Five a day for Health." Online. http://5aday.gov/index-about.shtml. Accessed November 25, 2003.

National Institutes of Health. *Clinical Guidelines on the Identification, Evaluation, and Treatment of Overweight and Obesity in Adults. The Evidence Report.* NIH Publication no. 98-4083; Sept 1998.

Nestle, M. *Food Politics.* Los Angeles: University of California Press, 2002.

Peek, P. *Fight Fat After Forty.* New York, NY: Viking Penguin, 2000.

Pinhas, L., B. Toner, B. Ali. "The Effects of the Ideal of Female Beauty on Mood and Body Satisfaction." *Int J Eat Disord* (1999).

Putnam, J., J. Allshouse, and L. Kantor. "U.S. per Capita Food Supply Trends: More Calories, Refined Carbohydrates, and Fats." *FoodReview* 25 (2002): 2-15.

Schneider M. "Listening to the Body: The Language of Stress-Related Symptoms." Workshop. Cortext Mind Matters, June 2001.

Shisslak, C. M., M. Crago, and L. S. Estes. "The Spectrum of Eating Disturbances." *Inter J Eat Dis* (1995).

U.S. Central Intelligence Agency. *The World Factbook.* Updated December 18, 2003. Available at: http://www.cia.gov/cia/publications/factbook/geos/us.html# Econ. Accessed March 22, 2004.

U.S. Department of Health and Human Services. *Physical Activity and Health: A Report of the Surgeon General.* Atlanta, GA: U.S. Department of Health and Human Services, Centers for Chronic Disease Prevention and Health Promotion, 1996.

U.S. Department of Health and Human Services. *Physical Activity Evaluation Handbook.* Atlanta, GA: U.S. Department of Health and Human Services, Centers for Chronic Disease Prevention and Health Promotion, 2002.

U.S. Department of Health and Human Services. *The Surgeon General's call to action to prevent and decrease overweight and obesity.* Washington, DC: U.S. Department of Health and Human Services, Public Health Services, Office of the Surgeon General, 2001.

Chapter Two

Carlson L. "Mindfulness-based Stress Reduction in Relation to Quality of Life, Mood, Symptoms of Stress and Levels of Cortisol, Dehydroepiandrosterone Sulfate(DHEAS) and Melatonin in Breast and Prostate Cancer Outpatients." *Psychoneuroendocrinology* (May 2004).

Cheikin, M. *An Integrated Medical Yoga Curriculum.* Workshop and notes presented at Kripalu Center for Yoga and Health, November 3-8, 2002, Lenox, MA.

Davidson, R., and J. Kabit-Zinn. "Alterations in Brain and Immune Function Produced by Mindfulness Meditation." *Psychosom Med* (Jul 2003).

Farhi, D. *Yoga Mind, Body and Spirit.* New York, NY: Henry Holt and Company, 2000.

Feuerstein, G. *The Yoga Tradition.* Prescott, AZ: Hohm Press, 1998.

Hartranft, C. *The Yoga Stra of Patañjali: Jewel of the Yoga Tradition.* Workshop and notes presented at The Arlington Center, June 2003, Arlington, MA.

Iyengar, B. K. S. *Light on Yoga.* New York, NY: Shocken Books, 1979.

Kripalu Yoga Fellowship. *Kripalu Yoga Teacher Training Manual.* Kripalu Center for Yoga and Health. Lenox, MA: 1998.

Rappaport, J. *365 Yoga Daily Meditations.* New York, NY: Penguin Group, 2002.

Seeman, T. "Religiosity/Spirituality and Health. A Critical Review of the Evidence for Biological Pathways." *Am Psychol* (Jan 2003).

Stoler Miller, B. *Yoga: Discipline of Freedom, the Yoga Sutra Attributed to Patanjali.* Berkeley, CA: University of California Press, 1995.

Chapter Three

Chödrön, P. Shambhala International. Halifax, Nova Scotia,Canada.

Dahlberg, C. "Living Large." *Yoga Journal* (December 2003).

Goldberg, M. "Intentional Yoga…On and Off the Mat." *Kripalu Yoga Teachers' Association Newsletter* (Spring 2000).

Rosal, M. "Facilitating Dietary Change: The Patient-Centered Counseling Model." *J Am Diet Assoc* (2001).

Chapter Four

Berg, F. *Children and Teens Afraid to Eat: Helping Youth in Today's Weight-Obsessed World.* Healthy Weight Network, 1997.

Cope, S. *Yoga and the Quest for the True Self.* New York, NY: Bantam Books, 1999.

Eifert, G., and M. Heffner. "The Effects of Acceptance Versus Control Contexts on Avoidance of Panic-Related Symptoms." *J Behav Ther Exp Psychiatry* (Sept 2003).

Hartranft, C. *The Yoga Sutras of Patanjali.* Boston, MA: Shambhala Publications, 2003.

Ladinsky, D. *The Gift—Poems by Hafiz.* New York, NY: Penguin Putnam, 1999.

LeShan, L. *Meditating to Attain a Healthy Weight.* New York, NY: Bantam, 1995.

Ritz, T., and M. Thons. "Airway Response of Healthy Individuals to Affective Picture Series." *Int J Psychophysiol* (Oct 2002).

S. Rama, R. Ballentine, and A. Hymes. *Science of Breath: A Practical Guide.* Fourth Printing. Honesdale, PA: The Himalayan Institute Press, 1998.

van den Wittenboer, G., K. van der Wolf, and J. van Dixhoorn. "Respiratory Variability and Psychological Well-Being in Schoolchildren." *Behav Modif* (Oct 2003).

van Diest, I., W. Winters, S. Devriese. "Hyperventilation Beyond Fight/Flight: Respiratory Responses During Emotional Imagery." *Psychophysiology* (Nov 2001).

Chapter Five

Benson, H., and E. Stuart. *The Wellness Book.* New York, NY: Simon & Schuster, 1992.

Elder J., G. Ayala, and S. Harris. "Theories and Intervention Approaches to Health-Behavior Change in Primary Care." *Am J Prev Med* (1999).

Hume, R. Translation. *The Thirteen Principal Upanishads*. London: The Oxford University Press, 1921.

Johnson, S. *Who Moved My Cheese?* New York, NY: Putnam, 1998.

National Institutes for Health. *Theory at a Glance: A Guide for Health Promotion Practice*. July 1995.

Prochaska, J., J. Norcross, and C. DiClemente. *Changing for Good: A Revolutionary Six-Stage Program for Overcoming Bad Habits and Moving Your Life Positively Forward*. New York, NY: Avon Books, 1994.

Winnett, R. "A Framework for Health Promotion and Disease Prevention Projects." *Am Psych* (1995).

Chapter Six

Blake, W. *There Is No Natural Religion*. Edited by M. Eaves, R. Essick, and J. Viscomi. The Institute for Advanced Technology in the Humanities. www.blakearchive.org. 1996-2002.

Wave Work Fellowship. Accessed at www.wavework.com. Accessed May 22, 2004.

Chapter Seven

Bland, J., E. Barrager, R. Reedy, and K. Bland. "A Medical Food-Supplemented Detoxification Program in the Management of Chronic Health Problems." *Altern Ther Health Med* (Nov 1995).

Health Services at Columbia University. Online. www.goaskalice.columbia.org. Accessed May 30, 2004.

Klapow, J., M. Slater, and T. Patterson. "Psychosocial Factors Discriminate Multidimensional Clinical Groups of Chronic Low Back Pain Patients." *Pain* (Sep 1995).

Percival, M. "Nutrition Support for Detoxification: Applied Nutritional Science Reports." *Advanced Nutrition Publications* (1997).

Robinson, R., Y. Murata, and K. Shimoda. "Dimensions of Social Impairment and Their Effect on Depression and Recovery Following Stroke." *Int Psychogeriatr* (Dec 1990).

U.S. Environmental Protection Agency. Office of Toxic Substances, Washington, DC. 2002 *Toxics Release Inventory (TRI)*. Public Data Release Report EPA260-R-04-003. June 2004.

Epilogue

Gibran, K. *The Prophet*. New York, NY: Knopf, 1923.

resources
for further study

Nutrition and Lifestyle Self-Assessment Tools

Aim for a Healthy Weight
National Heart, Lung, and Blood Institute
http://www.nhlbi.nih.gov/health/public/heart/obesity/lose_wt/index.htm

- Interactive BMI Calculator
- Interactive Menu Planner
- Information on Portion vs. Serving Size

Food Guide Pyramid
U.S. Department of Agriculture
http://mypyramid.gov

- Interactive help with foods and amounts right for you
- Interactive "my pyramid tracker" helps you assess and track your energy balance equation

Nutrition Information

American Dietetic Association (ADA)

www.eatright.org

- ❧ Find a dietitian in your area
- ❧ Fact sheets and nutrition information

Liz Lipski, PhD, CCN

www.innovativehealing.com

- ❧ Free library of articles from the complementary and alternative nutrition perspective
- ❧ Information on Dr. Lipski's workshops and services

Produce for Better Health Foundation

www.5aday.com

- ❧ Recipes and ideas for including fruits and vegetables in your diet
- ❧ Interactive "5aday" tracker

U.S. Department of Health and Human Services

www.nutrition.gov

- ❧ Nutrition and food safety information and fact sheets
- ❧ Resources and links to government nutrition programs

Favorite Books and Resources

Cooking and Eating

Brody, Jane. *Jane Brody's Nutrition Book.* New York, NY: W.W. Norton & Co, 1981.

Epicurious. www.epicurious.com

- ❧ A compilation of great searchable recipes from culinary magazines

Lipski, Elizabeth. *Digestive Wellness*. New Cannan, CT: Keats Publishing, 1996.

Mindful Nutrition and Conscious Eating

Altman, David. *The Art of the Inner Meal: Eating as a Spiritual Path*. New York, NY: HarperCollins, 1999.

David, Marc. *Nourishing Wisdom: A Mind-Body Approach to Nutrition and Well-being*. New York, NY: Harmony Books, 1991.

David, Marc. *The Slow Down Diet: Eating for Pleasure, Energy, and Weight Loss*. Rochester, VT: Healing Arts Press, 2005.

Weight and Body Image

Hirschmann, Jane, and Carol Munter. *When Women Stop Hating Their Bodies: Free Yourself from Food and Weight Obsession*. New York, NY: Fawcett Columbine, 1995.

Waterhouse, Debra. *Outsmarting the Female Fat Cell*. New York, NY: Warner Books, 1993.

Wolf, Naomi. *The Beauty Myth: How Images of Beauty Are Used Against Women*. New York, NY: Anchor Books, 1991.

Breaking Free (Geneen Roth) www.geneenroth.com

HUGS International (Linda Omichinsky) www.hugs.com

International Size Acceptance Association. www.size-acceptance.org

Women's campaign to End Body Hatred (Jane Hirschmann, Carol Munter) www.overcomingovereating.com

Detoxification

Bland, Jeffrey. *Toxicity and Inner Cleansing*. New Cannan, CT: Keats Publishing, 1987.

Haas, Elson. *The Detox Diet*. Berkley, CA: Celestial Arts, 1996.

Lipski, Haas, and Bland. *Leaky Gut Syndrome*. New Cannan, CT: Keats Publishing, 1998.

Page, L. *Detoxification*. Carmel Valley, CA: Traditional Wisdom, 2002.

Institute for Function Medicine. (800) 228-0622; www.fxmed.com

Yoga and Meditation

Cope, Stephen. *Yoga and the Quest for the True Self*. New York, NY: Bantam Books, 1999.

Farhi, Donna. *Yoga Mind, Body and Spirit*. New York, NY: Avon Books, 2000.

Iyengar, B. K. S. *Light on Yoga*. New York, NY: Schocken Books, Inc., 1966.

LeShan, Lawrence. *Meditating to Attain a Healthy Body Weight*. New York, NY: Bantam Books, 1994.

Mehta, S. *Yoga: The Iyengar Way*. New York, NY: Alfred Knopf, 1990.

Saraswati, Swami Janakananda. *Experience Yoga Nidra: Guided Deep Relaxation*. (CD)

Shiffman, Eric. *Yoga: The Spirit and Practice of Moving into Stillness*. New York, NY: Pocket Books, 1996.

Yoga Centers Providing CDs, Workshops, and Other Resources

Barbara Benagh

www.theyogastudio.org

Kripalu Center for Yoga and Health

(800) 741-7353

www.kripalu.org

Yoga Alliance

(928) 541-0004

www.yogaalliance.org

Yoga Research and Education Center/ International Association of Yoga Therapists

www.iayt.org

Yoga and Other Resources for Working with Emotions

Marcia Goldberg

www.lifeworkseastwest.com

12-Step Programs

www.12step.org

The Wave Work Fellowship

www.wavework.com

permissions

The author and publisher are grateful to the following writers, think-ers, and publishers, who have graciously provided their permission for the use of copyrighted materials.

- Yama and Niyama Chart and Chapter Two lead quote, copyright Kripalu Center for Yoga & Health, Yoga Teacher Training Manual (2006). Printed with permission.

- Intention exercises: Reprinted from "Intentional Yoga On and Off the Mat" by Marcia Goldberg. Kripalu Yoga Teachers' Association Newsletter, Spring 2000. Reprints of Articles are available at www.lifeworkseastwest.com.

- "Now Is the Time" from the Penguin publication *The Gift, Poems by Hafiz*, copyright 1999 Daniel Ladinsky, used with his permission.

- Riding the Wave of Emotion or Sensation: Wave Work Fellowship. The Wave Work®. Used with permission from www.wavework.com.

Every effort has been made to contact publishers to obtain their consent for reproducing quotes requiring permission under current copyright law. In cases where no response has been forthcoming or where we were unable to trace the author or publisher's current ad-dress, we gladly offer to add a full acknowledgment in future editions of this work as soon as we have been notified.

Mention of specific companies, organizations, or individuals does not imply endorsement by the publisher, nor does it imply that those men-tioned endorse this book. Internet addresses and other contact information provided were accurate at the time *Every Bite Is Divine* went to press.

index

f denotes references to illustrations, tables, and charts.

www.anniebkay.com